Contemporary Diagnosis and Management of

Hypertension in African Americans®

Elijah Saunders, MD
Professor of Medicine (Cardiology)
Head, Section of Hypertension
University of Maryland School of Medicine
Baltimore, Maryland

Wallace R. Johnson, MD
Clinical Assistant Professor of Medicine
Section of Hypertension
University of Maryland School of Medicine
Baltimore, Maryland

First Edition

Published by Handbooks in Health Care Co.,
Newtown, Pennsylvania, USA

International Standard Book Number: 1-884065-71-6

Library of Congress Catalog Card Number: 2001089594

Web site: www.HHCbooks.com

Contents

Preface 6

Chapter 1
Introduction 9

Chapter 2
Genetics, Physiology, and Mechanisms of Hypertension in African Americans 16

Chapter 3
Hypertension and Related Cardiovascular Risk Factors in African Americans 24

Chapter 4
Target Organ Damage in Hypertensive African Americans 85

Chapter 5
Classification and Evaluation of Hypertensive Patients 107

Chapter 6
Treatment of Hypertension in African Americans 116

Chapter 7
Role of Community Programs in the Management of Hypertension in African Americans 139

Chapter 8
Prevention of Hypertension 141

Appendix
Selected Guidelines
of the JNC 7 Report 145

Index 150

This book has been prepared and is presented as a service to the medical community. The information provided reflects the knowledge, experience, and personal opinions of the authors, Elijah Saunders, MD, Head, Section of Hypertension, University of Maryland School of Medicine, Baltimore, and Wallace R. Johnson, MD, Clinical Assistant Professor of Medicine, Section of Hypertension, University of Maryland School of Medicine.

This book is not intended to replace or to be used as a substitute for the complete prescribing information prepared by each manufacturer for each drug. Because of possible variations in drug indications, in dosage information, in newly described toxicities, in drug/drug interactions, and in other items of importance, reference to such complete prescribing information is definitely recommended before any of the drugs discussed are used or prescribed.

Preface

This handbook, *Contemporary Diagnosis and Management of Hypertension in African Americans®*, is being published during a period of remarkable change in the field of hypertension. Its construction has been a monumental but rewarding task because many landmark observational studies and large clinical trials were published after a working draft had been completed. However, the *Seventh Report of the Joint National Committee on Prevention, Detection, Evaluation, and Treatment of High Blood Pressure* (JNC 7), highlights of which were published in May 2003, and which will be released in full in fall 2003, will probably have an unparalleled impact on hypertension management. As a result, the authors have made some modifications to the previously written text in order to incorporate the new guidelines proposed by the JNC 7 report. Readers should keep in mind as they progress through this handbook that the *Sixth Report of the Joint National Committee on Prevention, Detection, Evaluation, and Treatment of High Blood Pressure* (JNC 6) was originally used as the basis for much of the text.

The JNC 7 report differs from the JNC 6 report in several ways:

1. Microalbuminuria, physical inactivity, and obesity have been added to the list of cardiovascular risk factors.
2. Sleep apnea is now listed as an identifiable cause of hypertension rather than a disease merely associated with hypertension.

3. Individuals with a systolic blood pressure of 120 to 139 mm Hg or a diastolic blood pressure of 80 to 89 mm Hg are now considered prehypertensive and require health-promoting lifestyle modifications to prevent cardiovascular disease.

4. Diabetic patients and patients with chronic kidney disease have a goal blood pressure of 130/80 mm Hg instead of 130/85 mm Hg, as noted in the JNC 6 report.

5. Any patient with a drug-naïve blood pressure of greater than 160/100 mm Hg is considered to have stage 2 hypertension; the stage 3 designation noted in the JNC 6 report has been dropped.

6. The JNC 7 report emphasizes the fact that in adults older than 50 years, a systolic blood pressure of more than 140 mm Hg is a much more important cardiovascular risk factor than diastolic blood pressure.

7. Angiotensin-receptor blockers, angiotensin-converting enzyme inhibitors, β-blockers, calcium antagonists, aldosterone antagonists, and, especially, diuretics all have additional compelling indications not originally noted in the JNC 6 report. For cxample, angiotensin-receptor blockers are now strongly indicated for heart failure, diabetes, and chronic kidney disease. This drug class had no compelling indications in previous JNC reports.

8. Two-drug therapy can now be recommended as initial therapy if the blood pressure is more than 20/10 mm Hg above the goal pressure, and it is now widely appreciated that most hypertensive patients will require combination therapy to reach their target blood pressure.

More comprehensive tables listing risk factors and guidelines as presented in the JNC 7 report can be found in the appendix to this handbook.

The above list is a representative sample of the notable differences between the JNC 7 report and the JNC 6 report. The figures, tables, and references included in this handbook will assist readers who wish to pursue more in-depth research into the management of hypertension. The authors feel that the algorithm designed by the International Society on Hypertension in Blacks, which can be found in this handbook in Chapter 6, will also serve as a user-friendly guide to hypertension management for physicians, nurses, and other allied health professionals.

The time has come for a guide to help clinicians who manage difficult, high-risk hypertensive patients such as African Americans. We hope that this handbook will earn its place in daily clinical practice and influence others to consider devoting time and effort to this challenging but rewarding effort.

Selected Readings

1. Chobanian AV, Bakris GL, Black HR, et al: The Seventh Report of the Joint National Committee on Prevention, Detection, Evaluation, and Treatment of High Blood Pressure: the JNC 7 report. *JAMA* 2003;289:2560-2572.

2. The Sixth Report of the Joint National Committee on Prevention, Detection, Evaluation and Treatment of High Blood Pressure. *Arch Intern Med* 1997;157:2413-2446.

3. Douglas JG, Bakris GL, Epstein M, et al: Management of high blood pressure in African Americans: consensus statement of the Hypertension in African Americans Working Group of the International Society on Hypertension in Blacks. *Arch Intern Med* 2003;163:525-541.

Chapter 1

Introduction

More than 50 million people in the United States are estimated to have hypertension. However, African Americans are disproportionately represented in this number. In fact, 32.4% of African Americans have hypertension, compared to 23.3% of non-Hispanic whites. This makes the prevalence of hypertension in African Americans among the highest in target populations in the world.

Although the incidence and prevalence of hypertension increase with age in all populations, they are much greater for African Americans (Figure 1-1). The difference in the prevalence of hypertension in African Americans and whites seems to begin just after puberty, and persists throughout adult life. Hypertension becomes common in older African-American women, so much so that by 65 years of age, as many as 75% of African-American women are hypertensive compared to about 50% of white women in the same age group.

Compared to whites, hypertension in African Americans develops earlier in life, tends to be more severe, and results in more target organ damage. Moreover, because African Americans have higher rates of stage 2 hypertension (defined as blood pressure ≥ 160 mm Hg systolic or ≥ 100 mm Hg diastolic), they have more cardiovascular morbidity and mortality. This greater burden of hypertensive complications leads to an 80% higher stroke mortality rate, a 50% higher heart disease mortality rate, and a

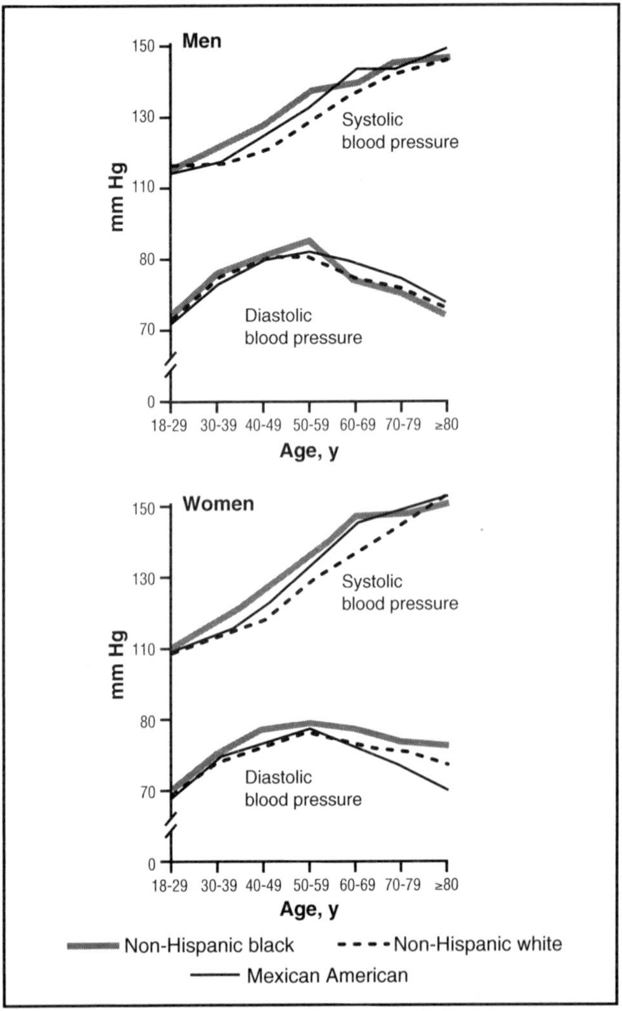

Figure1-1: Mean systolic and diastolic blood pressure by age and race/ethnicity for men and women 18 years of age and older, US population. Burt et al, *Hypertension* 1995;25:305-313.

320% higher rate of hypertension-related end-stage renal disease than in the general population.

Despite these depressing statistics, data and clinical experience have shown that African Americans can achieve overall declines in blood pressure similar to those in whites and that they experience lower incidences of cardiovascular disease when they get access to care and treatment equal to that which whites receive. Figures 1-2 and 1-3 reflect these phenomena in data supplied from the Vital Statistics of the United States, National Center for Health Statistics. However, our clinical experiences and many studies in the African-American community indicate that African Americans often do not receive a diagnosis of and treatment for hypertension until long after the disease is established and target organ damage has occurred.

Recognizing the Problem

Because hypertension is treated so frequently in physicians' offices, we believe there is a need for a concise, user-friendly handbook on this subject, geared toward primary care practitioners. The fact that African Americans get this disease earlier in life and suffer more serious consequences makes a handbook concentrating on this population particularly pertinent.

We do not attempt to define African Americans or blacks in the strictest terms of race, recognizing that race or ethnicity cannot be attributed to genetics alone but involves a constellation of social, psychologic, economic, and other environmental factors. Thus, when we speak of the *profile* of the hypertensive African-American, we are referring to descriptors that occur more commonly in persons recognized or self-identified as being of African origin. Regardless of the definition, race is clearly a high-risk contributor to mortality in the hypertensive population. The diagnosis of hypertension is generally uncomplicated, and treatment is effective in preventing a high rate of disability and death in hypertensive African Americans as well as whites. Yet

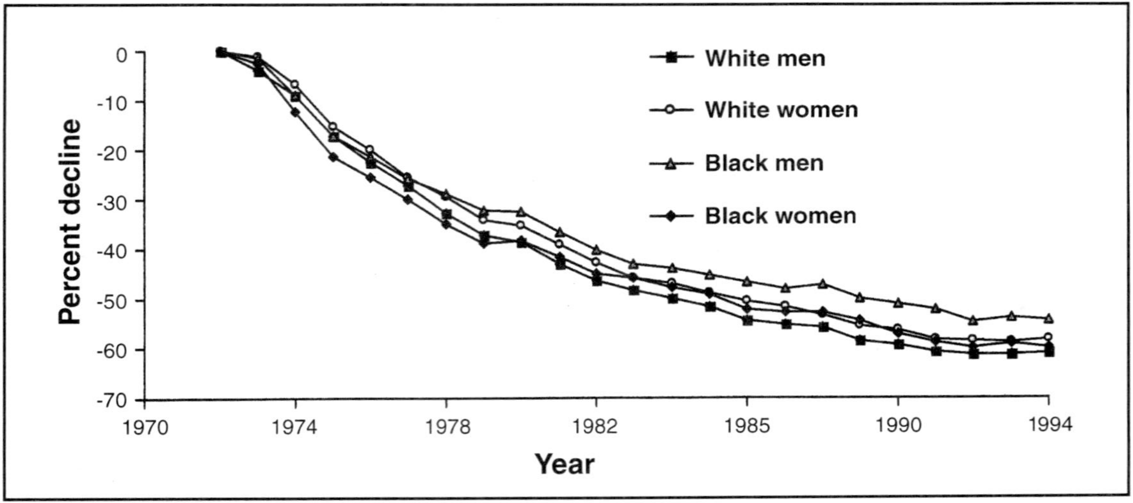

Figure 1-2: Percentage decline in age-adjusted mortality rates for stroke by sex and race, United States, 1972-1994. Prepared using data from Vital Statistics of the United States, National Center for Health Statistics. Age-adjusted to the 1940 US census population. The decline in age-adjusted mortality from stroke in the total population is 59%.

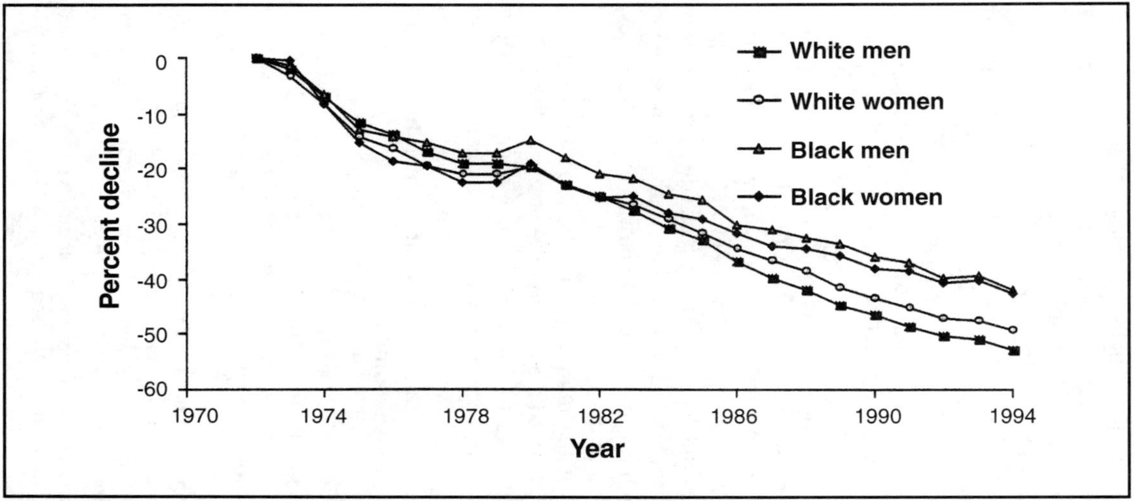

Figure 1-3: Percentage decline in age-adjusted mortality rates by sex and race for coronary heart disease, United States, 1972-1994. Prepared using data from Vital Statistics of the United States, National Center for Health Statistics. Age-adjusted to the 1940 US census population. The decline in age-adjusted mortality for coronary heart disease in the total population is 53.2%.

mortality from all forms of hypertension-related cardiovascular diseases remains disproportionately high in blacks compared to whites, despite the fact that studies show treatment benefits to be similar in both races.

In this handbook, we examine the epidemiology, physiology, and pathophysiology of hypertension in blacks, especially as they are related to management. We attempt to follow the national guidelines of the Joint National Committee on Prevention, Detection, Evaluation and Treatment of High Blood Pressure and evidence-based data, but we deviate slightly when preliminary data or our experience calls for the presentation of information that may have important implications for the African-American population. An important aspect of pharmacologic treatment of hypertension in African Americans is the racial difference in drug responsiveness. While we emphasize that hypertensive blacks and whites share more similarities than differences, those differences must be appreciated.

Because of the uniqueness of the African-American community, we find it useful to present some of the alternative approaches to the management of hypertension. Finally, our long-term experiences in the control of hypertension in various community settings persuade us to describe these programs and encourage their broader application in similar communities.

Selected Readings

Burt VL, Whelton P, Roccella EJ, et al: Prevalence of hypertension in the US adult population. Results from the Third National Health and Nutrition Examination Survey, 1988-1991. *Hypertension* 1995;25:305-313.

Five-year findings of the Hypertension and Follow-up Program: mortality by race, sex, and blood pressure level. A further analysis. Hypertension Detection and Follow-up Program Cooperative Group. *J Community Health* 1984;9:314-327.

Hall WD, Ferrario CM, Moore MA, et al: Hypertension-related morbidity and mortality in the southeastern United States. *Am J Med Sci* 1997;313:195-209.

Hildreth C, Saunders E: Hypertension in blacks: clinical overview. In: Saunders E, ed. *Cardiovascular Diseases in Blacks*. Philadelphia, FA Davis, 1991, pp 85-96.

Klag MJ, Whelton PK, Randall BL, et al: End-stage renal disease in African-American and white men. 16-year MRFIT findings. *JAMA* 1997;277:1293-1298.

Ooi WL, Budner NS, Cohen H, et al: Impact of race on treatment response and cardiovascular disease among hypertensives. *Hypertension* 1989;14:227-234.

Singh GK, Kochanek KD, MacDorman MF: Advance report of final mortality statistics, 1994. *Mon Vital Stat Rep* 1996;45(suppl 3):1-76.

Voors AW, Foster TA, Frerichs RR, et al: Studies of blood pressure in children, ages 5-14 years, in a total biracial community: the Bugalusa Heart Study. *Circulation* 1976;54:319-327.

Chapter **2**

Genetics, Physiology, and Mechanisms of Hypertension in African Americans

As with many chronic diseases, considerable debate exists about whether hypertension is caused by genetic aberrations or by environmental factors. Hypertension is so common in African Americans and in people of African descent living in Western and/or urban environments that it is typically explained by the contention that people of African descent "are *intrinsically susceptible* to high blood pressure because of some vaguely defined aspect of their genetic makeup." However, Cooper argues that this conclusion is not satisfying because it does not accurately reflect the available evidence. He points out that genetic variations in hypertension have been found more within races than between races. Although genetic studies have shown positive correlation between the renin-angiotensin-aldosterone system (RAAS) and hypertension, correlation with race has not been identified (Figure 2-1). The importance of an up-regulated RAAS, especially at the tissue level, may explain the high rate of target organ damage in many hypertensive patients, such as African Americans, and may have significant therapeutic implications. Target organ damage is examined in more detail in Chapter 4.

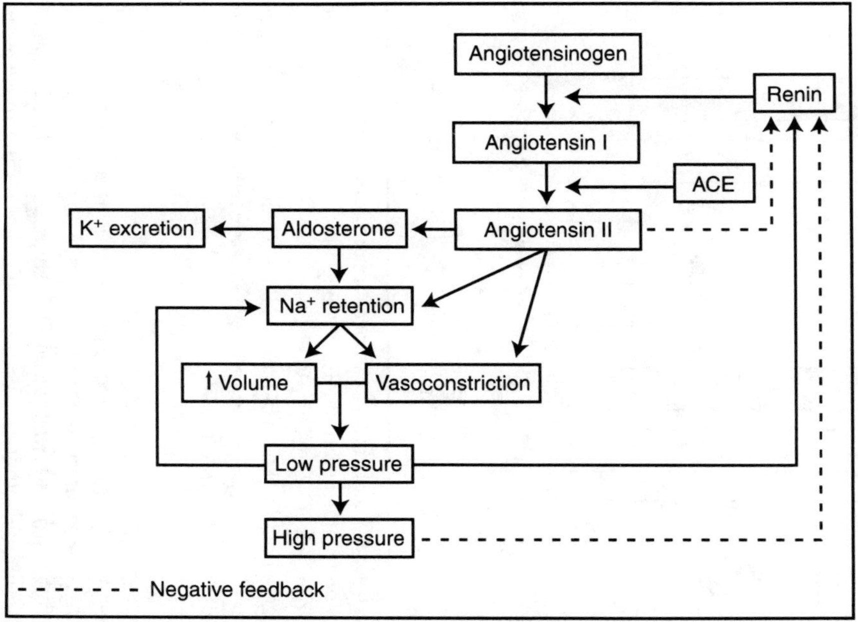

Figure 2-1: The circulating renin-angiotensin-aldosterone system (RAAS). This biochemical pathway influences blood pressure. People with a highly active RAAS typically have high blood pressure. ACE = angiotensin-converting enzyme. Adapted from Laragh JH: *Laragh's Lessons in Renin System Pathophysiology for Treating Hypertension and Its Fatal Cardiovascular Consequences.* New York, Elsevier Science Inc, 2002. Cover.

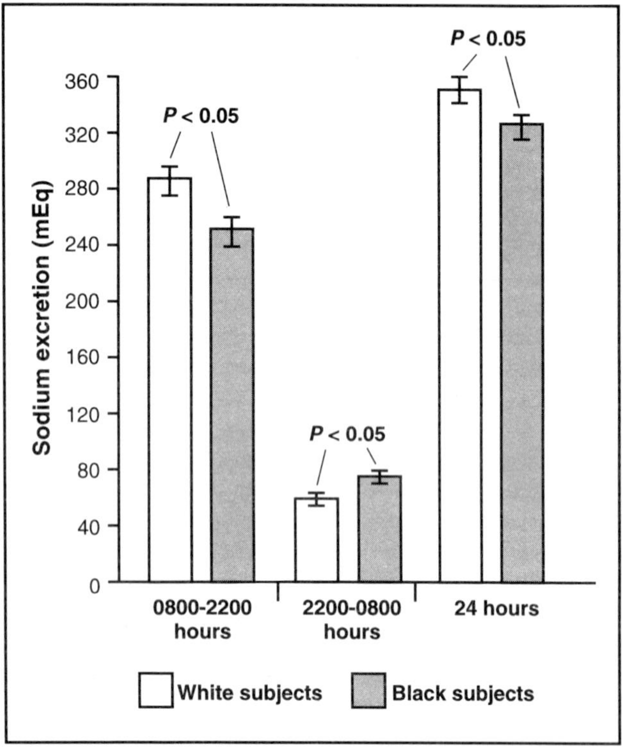

Figure 2-2: Urinary sodium excretion during volume expansion of matched normal white and black subjects. Reprinted from Luft FC, Grim CE, Weinberger MH: Electrolyte and volume homeostasis in blacks. In Hall WD, Saunders E, Shulman NB, eds: *Hypertension in Blacks: Epidemiology, Pathophysiology, and Treatment*. Chicago: Mosby-Year Book, 1985, pp 119-120, with permission from Elsevier Science.

One frequently cited explanation for the increased rate of hypertension in African Americans is based on the voyage from Africa to America on slave ships (the Middle Passage). Grim and others have speculated that during these ardu-

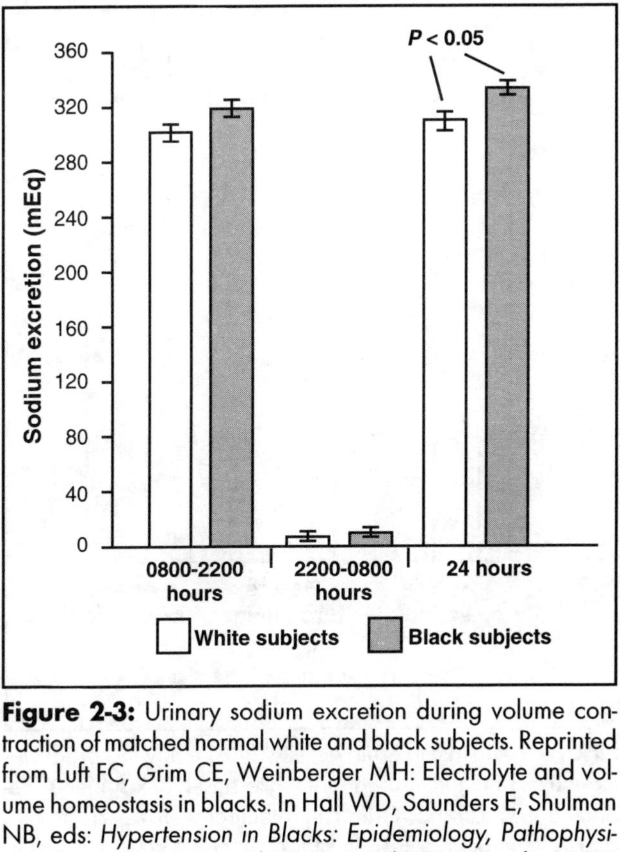

Figure 2-3: Urinary sodium excretion during volume contraction of matched normal white and black subjects. Reprinted from Luft FC, Grim CE, Weinberger MH: Electrolyte and volume homeostasis in blacks. In Hall WD, Saunders E, Shulman NB, eds: *Hypertension in Blacks: Epidemiology, Pathophysiology, and Treatment*. Chicago: Mosby-Year Book, 1985, pp 119-120, with permission from Elsevier Science.

ous trips, the slaves were placed in a Darwinian 'survival of the fittest' situation, in which survival depended on 'high-sodium-retaining' genes. Once an individual with these genes assumed a lifestyle in an environment in which sodium was plentiful (acculturation), the hypothesis suggests, the risk of hypertension escalated. This theory remains controversial.

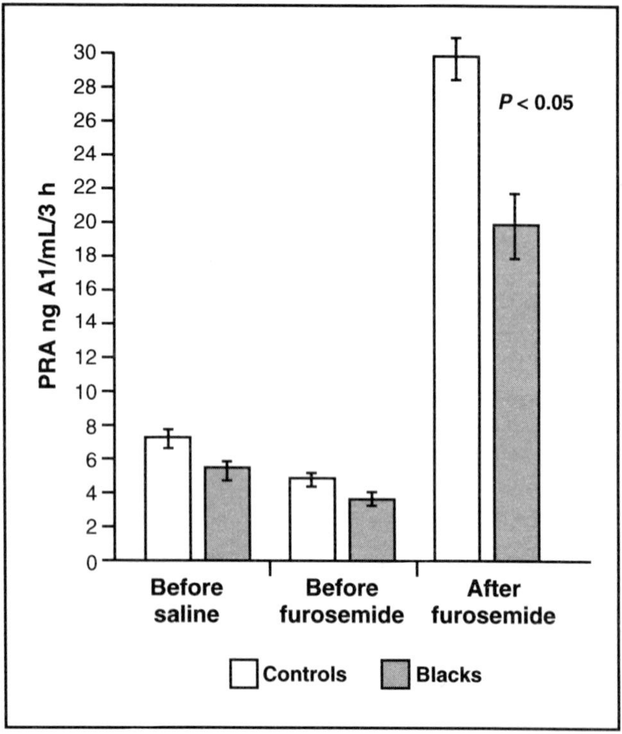

Figure 2-4: Plasma renin activity (PRA) following proactive maneuvers in matched normal white and black subjects. Reprinted from Luft FC, Grim CE, Weinberger MH: Electrolyte and volume homeostasis in blacks. In Hall WD, Saunders E, Shulman NB, eds: *Hypertension in Blacks: Epidemiology, Pathophysiology, and Treatment*. Chicago: Mosby-Year Book, 1985, pp 119-120, with permission from Elsevier Science.

Physiologically, blood pressure is a function of cardiac output and systemic vascular resistance. Researchers believe that early in the development of hypertension, cardiac output is the predominant factor, but systemic vascular resistance is responsible for the maintenance of high blood pressure in established hypertension. The role that sodium plays in expanding plasma volume and the role of the kidneys in regulating sodium homeostasis have been well described. Certain features have been demonstrated to be different in African Americans than in whites, which may explain the pathogenesis of excessive target organ damage and the higher mortality in hypertensive African Americans. This is particularly true for stroke, for which morbidity and mortality are excessive in African Americans but can be reduced significantly by treating blood pressure. Many studies support the following profile of the hypertensive African American:

- Low plasma renin activity and renin hypersensitivity
- Increased sodium sensitivity and possible plasma volume expansion; Figures 2-2, 2-3, and 2-4 demonstrate significant differences in sodium handling and plasma renin activity in black and white patients
- Lower kallikrein and prostaglandin levels
- Greater sensitivity to the pressor effects of norepinephrine and lower levels of dopamine β-hydroxylase
- Greater vascular reactivity to stressors such as cold pressor test and mental arithmetic
- Increased insulin resistance
- Higher nocturnal blood pressures
- Probable increased levels of endothelin, vasoconstrictor receptors, and growth receptors
- Possible lower levels of natriuretic peptides and higher levels of ouabain-like sodium pump inhibitor

The role of potassium in hypertension, especially in blacks, seems to be a protective one. Blacks have been shown to ingest less potassium, contributing to a greater sodium/potassium ratio in the urine, which correlates with higher blood pressure levels. Data have shown that potassium may mitigate the adverse effect of sodium on blood pressure and vascular damage. Epidemiologic and experimental studies have supported these observations. A clinical study done in California demonstrated a significant relationship between dietary potassium and subsequent stroke mortality. A more recent study and the results of the Dietary Approaches to Stop Hypertension (DASH) diet trials have helped to confirm the beneficial role of potassium in hypertension. The roles of calcium and magnesium are still being studied. Elevated insulin levels and insulin resistance associated with hypertension are also suspected to be more common in African Americans.

Selected Readings

Blaustein MP, Grim CE: The pathogenesis of hypertension: black-white differences. In: Saunders E, Davis FA, eds. *Cardiovascular Diseases in Blacks*. Philadelphia, 1991, p 102.

Cooper RS: Cerebrovascular disease in blacks. In: Hall DW, Saunders E, Shulman NB, eds. *Hypertension in Blacks: Epidemiology, Pathophysiology, and Treatment*. Chicago, Year Book Medical Publishers, 1985, p 102.

Cooper RS, Kaufman JS: Race and hypertension: science and nescience. *Hypertension* 1998;32:813-816.

Cooper RS, Rotimi CN: Hypertension in populations of West African origin: is there a genetic predisposition? *J Hypertens* 1994; 12:215-227.

Cooper RS, Rotimi CN, Ataman SL, et al: Hypertension prevalence in seven populations of African origin. *J Public Health* 1997;87:160-168.

Dustan HP: Does keloid pathogenesis hold the key to understanding black/white differences in hypertension severity? *Hypertension* 1995;26(pt 1):858-862.

Fray JC: *Pathophysiology of Hypertension in Blacks*. New York, Oxford University Press, 1993, p 217.

Gretler DD, Fumo MT, Nelson KS, et al: Ethnic differences in circadian hemodynamic profile. *Am J Hypertens* 1994;7:7-14.

Grim CE, Wilson TW: Salt, slavery and survival: physiological principles underlying the evolutionary hypothesis of salt sensitivity hypertension in Western Hemisphere blacks. In: Fray JC, Douglass JG, eds. *Pathophysiology of Hypertension in Blacks*. New York, Oxford University Press, 1992.

Helmer OM: The renin-angiotensin system and its relation to hypertension. *Prog Cardiovasc Dis* 1965;8:117-128.

Khaw KT, Barrett-Conner E: Dietary potassium and stroke-associated mortality. A 12-year prospective population study. *N Engl J Med* 1987;316:235-240.

Kotanko P, Binder A, Tasker J, et al: Essential hypertension in African Caribbeans associates with a variant of the β_2-adrenoceptor. *Hypertension* 1997;30:773-776.

Luft FC, Grim CE, Weinberger MH: Electrolyte and volume homeostasis in blacks. In: Hall DW, Saunders E, Shulman NB, eds. *Hypertension in Blacks: Epidemiology, Pathophysiology, and Treatment*. Chicago, Year Book Medical Publishers, 1985, p 118.

Osei K, Cottrell DA: Minimal model analyses of insulin sensitivity and glucose-dependent glucose disposal in black and white Americans: a study of persons at risk for type 2 diabetes. *Eur J Clin Invest* 1994;24:843-850.

Saunders E: Hypertension in blacks. *Med Clin North Am* 1987; 71:1013-1029.

Song Q, Chao J, Chao L: DNA polymorphisms in the 5'-flanking region of the human tissue kallikrein gene. *Hum Genet* 1997; 996:727-734.

Tobian L, MacNeill D, Johnson MA, et al: Potassium protection against lesions of the renal tubules, arteries, and glomeruli and nephron loss in salt-loaded hypertensive Dahl S rats. *Hypertension* 1984;6(pt 2):1170-1176.

Weiss SJ: Editorial policies and practices. *J Clin Invest* 1998;101:6-7.

Woods JW, Falk RJ, Pittman AW, et al: Increased red-cell sodium-lithium countertransport in normotensive sons of hypertensive parents. *N Engl J Med* 1982;306:593-595.

Chapter **3**

Hypertension and Related Cardiovascular Risk Factors in African Americans

Obesity

The American Heart Association has classified obesity as a major modifiable risk factor for coronary artery disease. This comes as no surprise in the United States, where it is estimated that the indirect and direct health-care costs of obesity exceed $70 billion annually. In addition, major studies such as the National Health and Nutrition Examination Survey III (NHANES III), conducted between 1988 and 1994, have shown that 55% of the US population is overweight and that 22.5% is obese. The terms *overweight* and *obese* are defined in Table 3-1.

The incidence of obesity has been increasing in all racial/ethnic, gender, and age groups and is extensive in African Americans, with 65.9% of women and 56.7% of men classified as overweight or obese, according to the NHANES III data. The same study classified 60.6% of white men and 47% of white women as overweight or obese.

The regulation and maintenance of body weight are complex and not fully understood, involving appetite control, genetics, and physiology. Thus, despite the fact that approximately $40 billion is spent on weight loss treatment each year in the United States alone, the incidence of obesity has not decreased. One reason is that as the obese person decreases his or her body weight, the body responds by decreasing energy expenditure. In fact, for every 10% drop in body weight, there is a 25% drop in energy expenditure. This may explain why many weight loss programs are unsuccessful.

In 1967, the Framingham Heart Study demonstrated that increased body weight is associated with increased blood pressure. In fact, in the Framingham study population, investigators found that 70% of new hypertension patients were obese. Furthermore, epidemiologic studies indicate that one third of hypertension incidence is related to obesity and that obese patients are three times more likely to develop hypertension than their lean counterparts. Fortunately, both systolic and diastolic blood pressure can be reduced through weight loss. A modest weight reduction of 5% to 10% has been shown to significantly reduce blood pressure. However, studies have also found that most obese persons do not sustain their weight loss for more than 5 years. How, then, should the practicing health care provider treat obesity and corresponding hypertension? Initially, both the patient and the physician must agree on a realistic goal, such as a 10% decrease in body weight over 6 to 9 months.

More specifically, it is important to consider how obesity relates to hypertension. The Framingham Study discovered that for every 10-pound weight gain there was a 4.5-mm Hg increase in systolic blood pressure. Although some physicians attributed the hypertension to poor eating habits (ie, high-salt, high-fat diets), at least one large study has found obesity to be strongly associated with high blood pressure independent of sodium or potassium intake. Increased potassium intake appears to mitigate the adverse effects of sodium on blood pressure and vascular damage, according to epidemiologic and experimental studies. Therefore, it is likely that other mechanisms are

Table 3-1: Classification of Overweight and Obesity by BMI, Waist Circumference, and Associated Disease Risks*

	BMI (kg/m²)	Obesity Class
Underweight	< 18.5	
Normal	18.5-24.9	
Overweight	25.0-29.9	
Obesity	30.0-34.9	I
	35.0-39.9	II
Extreme Obesity	≥ 40	III

BMI = body mass index

*Disease risk relative to normal weight and waist circumference

responsible for obesity-induced hypertension. Recently, the insulin resistance syndrome has been implicated as the major mechanism for obesity-induced blood pressure. The syndrome is characterized by high plasma insulin levels, dyslipidemia, android obesity, and hypertension. The higher insulin levels appear to cause sodium retention, increased sympathetic nervous system activity, and vascular hypertrophy, all of which contribute to hypertension. Lean hypertensive patients can also develop insulin resistance syndrome, but it is much more common in obese hypertensive patients. Insulin resistance syndrome is often associated with type 2 diabetes and is frequently found in those with upper-body obesity. There is no specific treatment for insulin resistance syndrome, but all patients should try to achieve good control of their glucose, lipids,

Men ≤ 102 cm (≤ 40 in) Women ≤ 88 cm (≤ 35 in)	Men > 102 cm (> 40 in) Women > 88 cm (> 35 in)
—	—
—	—
Increased	High
High	Very high
Very high	Very high
Extremely high	Extremely high

Coleman, *ABC Digest Urban Cardiology* 1999;6:23-28.

blood pressure, and weight. Drugs such as metformin (Glucophage®) and the glitazones (pioglitazone [Actos®], rosiglitazone [Avandia®]) are insulin sensitizers, which have also been shown to lower blood pressure and therefore should be considered for insulin-resistant patients. Insulin sensitizers act to increase the sensibility of skeletal muscle to the action of insulin, thus increasing glucose uptake into skeletal muscle. More information on this subject is found in the section on insulin resistance in this chapter.

The mechanism by which obesity induces hypertension is likely multifactorial, involving increased sympathetic nervous system activation, enhanced renal sodium and water retention, and impaired vasodilatation, which could be a result of high insulin levels and/or dyslipidemia. The best treatment for obesity-induced hypertension is cer-

Table 3-2: Agents for the Management of Obesity

Category	Pharmacologic Class	Agents
Appetite Suppressants	Centrally acting adrenergic agents	Benzphetamine, phendimetrazine, diethylpropion, mazindol
	Nonadrenergic agents	Phentermine
	Serotoninergic agents	Fenfluramine,* dexfenfluramine,* fluoxetine,** sertraline**
	Adrenergic/ serotoninergic agents	Sibutramine
Thermogenic Agents	Adrenergic agents	Ephedrine/caffeine combination
	β_3 agonists†	Not commercially available BRL 26830A, BRL 35135, CL 316243, RO 40-2148, RO 16-8714, ZD 7114

tainly weight loss, but, unfortunately, successful weight loss is hard to maintain in many patients. Therefore, many clinicians must content themselves with treating the risk factors induced by obesity or prescribing one of the anti-obesity drugs on the market (Table 3-2).

Category	Pharmacologic Class	Agents
Hormonal Manipulation	Leptin analogs, neuropeptide Y antagonists[†]	Not commercially available
Digestive Inhibitors	Lipase inhibitors	Orlistat
	Fat substitutes:	
	Carbohydrate based	N/A
	Protein based	N/A
	Fat based	Olestra

*Withdrawn from the US market in September 1997

**Not FDA approved for the treatment of obesity

[†]Investigational drugs

Coleman, *ABC Digest Urban Cardiology* 1999;6:23-28.

No consensus exists on how we should treat obesity, but most practitioners favor a multifaceted approach that includes diet, exercise, behavior modification, and, in the more difficult cases, drug therapy. Because obesity is so difficult to treat, we must target overweight adoles-

Table 3-3: Major Contraindications to Antiobesity Medications

- Recent stroke (within 3 years)
- Uncontrolled hypertension
- Unstable cardiovascular disease (angina pectoris)
- General anesthesia

cents before they go on to develop class I obesity. Furthermore, in the African-American community, we must develop ways to encourage exercise, such as church-sponsored aerobics, walking clubs, and more gym activities in city schools. For patients requiring pharmacologic treatment, we must be careful not to let a strong desire to treat obesity override safety concerns (Table 3-3). This is especially true because some antiobesity agents (ie, phentermine, sibutramine [Meridia®, Reductil®]) can cause acute hypertension.

Table 3-2 lists antiobesity agents, but clinicians must remember that only three are approved by the US Food and Drug Administration (FDA): sibutramine, phentermine, and orlistat (Xenical®). However, before using any of these agents, clinicians should emphasize to patients that drug therapy is an adjunct to diet and exercise. Also, physicians should screen patients for depression and thyroid disease, which can impede weight-loss efforts. If depression must be treated, clinicians should consider bupropion (Wellbutrin®, Zyban®), which can sometimes lead to modest weight loss. Alternatively, a serotonin (5-HT) antidepressant such as nefazodone (Serzone®) or an antidepressant such as venlafaxine (Effexor®) can be used.

Sibutramine, a relatively new antiobesity drug as effective as other drugs on the market, has been found to cause a dose-dependent increase in blood pressure of 3 to 4 mm Hg in both systolic and diastolic pressures. Phentermine is an older, less costly antiobesity agent, but it is relatively contraindicated in patients with coronary artery disease and/or moderate hypertension. Sibutramine is more expensive than phentermine but may have a lesser hypertensive effect; clinically significant increases in blood pressure occurred in less than 5% of the studied population. Sibutramine costs approximately $3 per pill and often is not fully effective until 6 months or more of therapy, which is a major limitation to its use.

Orlistat received FDA approval in 1999. It acts to reduce weight by inhibiting gastric and pancreatic lipases, thereby blocking a significant portion of dietary fat absorption. Orlistat is given as a 120-mg dose with meals and has been found to be effective in clinical trials in inducing weight loss irrespective of meal composition. Most of the adverse effects are gastrointestinal, including abdominal bloating, loose stools, flatulence, and anal leak. However, reducing fat consumption often significantly reduces these side effects.

While the search continues for better antiobesity therapy, clinicians should promote diet and exercise while aggressively treating comorbid cardiovascular disease. Patients who are resistant to lifestyle changes alone can use adjunctive pharmacologic therapy as long as the benefits exceed the risks.

Obesity and Sleep Apnea

Sleep apnea and sleep disordered breathing (SDB) have been associated with hypertension in clinical studies. Most studies using polysomnography found an association between sleep apnea and hypertension independent of age, sex, weight, and other potential confounding variables. In the largest study on sleep apnea published to date, the authors found a high prevalence of apneic events across racial and ethnic groups, as well as a clear association between the increasing frequency of apneic events and hypertension. However, the authors point out that an association between apneic events and hypertension does not definitely prove a causal relationship.

There is increasing evidence that untreated sleep apnea induces sustained arterial hypertension. This hypertension is thought to be secondary to sympathetic nervous system excitation, which results in elevated catecholamine levels in the bloodstream. However, the elevated plasma and urine catecholamine levels are not present during apnea-free periods. Therefore, sustained hypertension during wakefulness is not fully explained by the surge in sympathetic activity. Variables such as obesity, sex, alcohol, and smoking can also have a parallel impact on the frequency of apnea and cause hypertension through separate mechanisms.

What are the treatment implications of correlating sleep apnea to hypertension? Continuous positive airway pressure (CPAP) therapy reduces apneic events and often results in improvement in blood pressure during wakefulness. The diagnosis of sleep-apnea-induced hypertension can be especially difficult in African Americans because the incidence of essential hypertension is higher in this population. Thus, a trial of CPAP therapy seems prudent in appropriate patients, especially since African Americans also have a higher incidence of resistant hypertension. It is important for clinicians to evaluate at-risk patients, such as obese patients, loud-snoring patients, patients with witnessed apneic events, and patients with resistant hypertension. Overall, CPAP therapy seems to have good potential benefits with no significant adverse effects, although cost and inconvenience are issues.

Unfortunately, many clinicians do not look for obstructive sleep apnea unless the patient has the classic pickwickian syndrome, which is sleep apnea associated with morbid obesity, daytime somnolence, chronic hypercapnia, and hypoxemia. The typical obstructive sleep apnea patient is a man, 30 to 60 years of age, who has a history of snoring, daytime sleepiness, only moderate obesity, and mild to moderate hypertension. Therefore, it is important to consider the diagnosis of obstructive sleep apnea in any patient with resistant hypertension.

Take-home Points on Obesity

- Clinicians should know the National Institutes of Health (NIH) guidelines on obesity.
- Fat accumulation in the abdomen seems to increase cardiac risk, independent of being overweight.
- Many patients who lose weight will regain it in 3 to 5 years.
- Clinicians should encourage patients to avoid 'yo-yo' dieting (rapid increases and decreases in weight).
- Clinicians should encourage low, gradual weight loss based on each patient's needs.
- The following is the suggested formula for losing 1 pound per week: [weight (in lb) x 13 kcal] - 500 kcal = daily caloric requirement.
- All obese patients should exercise, unless there is a definite contraindication.
- Pharmacologic agents (Table 3-2) should be considered if the risk of obesity exceeds the potential health risk of the antiobesity agent.
- A review of 11 studies found that a 1-kg (2.2-lb) decrease in body weight corresponded with a 1.6-mm Hg systolic and 1.3-mm Hg diastolic reduction in blood pressure.
- Weight loss often reduces the number of antihypertensive agents needed.
- Weight loss may reduce left ventricular mass.

Diabetes Mellitus

Diabetes mellitus is clearly one of the most serious diseases affecting the African-American population. In 1998, diabetes was diagnosed in 1.5 million African Americans, representing a fourfold increase over the incidence in 1968. Moreover, an estimated 700,000 African Americans have diabetes and do not know it. Diabetes is more prevalent among African Americans than among whites; in fact, for every 6 white Americans who have diabetes, 10 African-Americans have the disease. Also, the incidence of diabetes increases with age. Among African Americans aged 50 years and older, 19% of men and 28% of women have diabetes. Moreover, African Americans with diabetes are more likely to develop complications and have greater diabetes-related disability than whites. For example, according to the NHANES III data, African Americans have a frequency of diabetic retinopathy that is 40% higher than that in whites, while diabetic end-stage renal disease is 4 times higher. African Americans have a 27% higher mortality rate related to diabetes compared to whites.

Most African Americans with diabetes have type 2 diabetes; only 5% to 10% have type 1 diabetes. Unfortunately, an increasing number of US adolescents are developing type 2 diabetes, probably as a result of the increasing rate of obesity in America. Investigators are aggressively studying how to prevent obesity and its associated diabetes, and why a higher rate of hypertension exists in the obese adolescent population. Clinicians are also concerned about what will happen to these obese adolescents when they become adults and whether they will develop complications at an even earlier age than seen in the past.

Clinicians and researchers know that diabetes and hypertension frequently occur together. Fortunately, the treatment for one (specifically weight reduction, increased physical activity, sodium restriction, and moderation of alcohol intake) helps control the other. The *Seventh Report of the Joint National Committee on Prevention, Detection, Evaluation, and Treatment of High Blood Pressure* (JNC 7) set a goal blood pressure of less than 130/80 mm Hg for patients with diabetes or chronic kidney disease. The American Diabetes Association and the National

Kidney Foundation state that diabetic patients should reach a minimum blood pressure of 130/80 mm Hg. Because most diabetic, hypertensive patients, particularly African Americans, will need more than one antihypertensive agent to reach goal blood pressure, clinicians must know which agents should be used as first-line therapy, based on available clinical trials (Figure 3-1).

The results of recent clinical trials, such as the Fosinopril Versus Amlodipine Cardiovascular Events Randomized Trial (FACET) and the Appropriate Blood Pressure Control in Diabetes (ABCD) trial, leave little doubt that angiotensin-converting enzyme (ACE) inhibitors should be strongly considered as first-line therapy in hypertensive patients with diabetes, especially if proteinuria is present. In addition, recent clinical trials in hypertensive patients with type 2 diabetes found that angiotensin-receptor blockers (ARBs) are effective in protecting against further progression of nephropathy and that this protection is independent of the effect of blood pressure control. The Irbesartan Diabetic Nephropathy Trial (IDNT) found that the ARB irbesartan (Avapro®) had renoprotective effects in patients with type 2 diabetes. These effects were significantly better than those found with amlodipine (Norvasc®) or conventional antihypertensive agents. Moreover, the Reduction of Endpoints in NIDDM with the Angiotensin II Antagonist Losartan (RENAAL) study found that losartan (Cozaar®) significantly protects against the progression of nephropathy in patients with type 2 diabetes compared with that found with conventional antihypertensive agents. In the Irbesartan Microalbuminuria Type 2 Diabetes in Hypertensive Patients Study (IRMA-2), irbesartan significantly reduced nephropathy in diabetic patients with microalbuminuria and slowed progression from microalbuminuria to overt proteinuria.

Many clinicians do not realize that while ACE inhibitors have been shown to be preferred to calcium-channel blockers in reducing cardiovascular events, the subset of

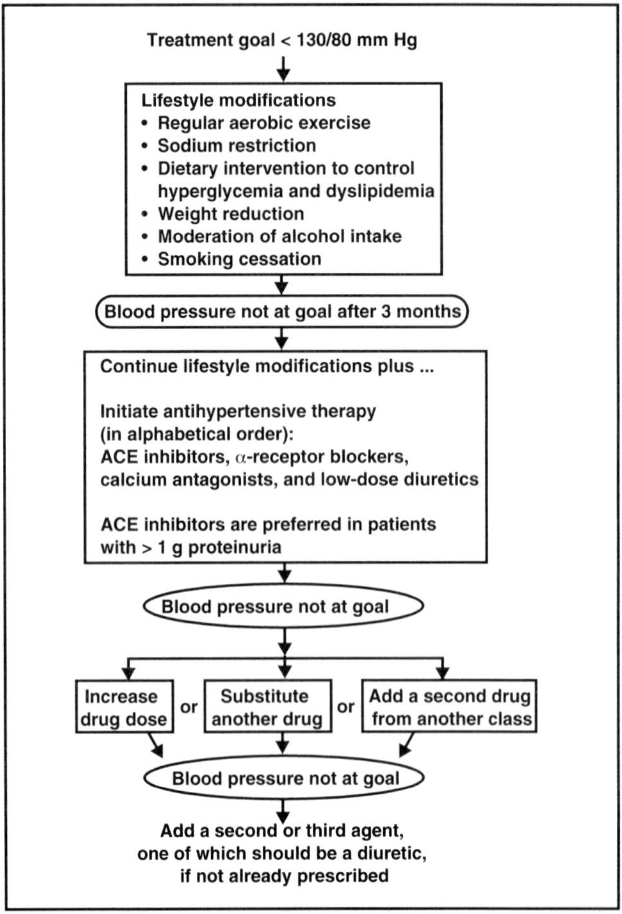

Figure 3-1: Treatment of diabetic, hypertensive patients. ACE = angiotensin-converting enzyme. Modified from Sowers, *J Clin Hypertens (Greenwich)* 1999;1:41-47. Reproduced with permission from LeJacq Communications, Inc. Note: Recommendations from the American Diabetes Association and National Kidney Foundation state that the blood pressure goal should be 130/80 mm Hg or less.

patients taking both ACE inhibitors and calcium-channel blockers did better than those taking either agent alone in the FACET trial. The FACET and ABCD trials each used a dihydropyridine calcium-channel blocker, amlodipine and nisoldipine (Sular®), respectively. It would be interesting to conduct similar trials with nondihydropyridine calcium antagonists to see if the same findings would occur, especially to determine if an ACE inhibitor/diuretic combination would reduce the incidence of nephropathy more than an ACE inhibitor/nondihydropyridine calcium-antagonist combination.

Thiazide diuretics and β-blockers were used less frequently in the 1980s after clinicians became concerned about drug-induced metabolic problems. However, in the Systolic Hypertension in the Elderly Program (SHEP) study, patients with type 2 diabetes, especially elderly men who received diuretics and β-blockers, derived as much benefit in terms of coronary disease and stroke reduction as nondiabetic patients, even when diuretics and β-blockers were used in the nondiabetic group.

Thiazide diuretics in low doses (< 25 mg of hydrochlorothiazide [Esidrix®, HydroDIURIL®, Microzide®, Oretic®] or chlorthalidone [Hygroton®, Thalitone®] daily) often have good efficacy without causing significant metabolic abnormalities. Combination therapy using diuretics and ACE inhibitors has become popular, especially because it results in even greater blood pressure reduction than either agent used alone, and the addition of an ACE inhibitor further minimizes the potential for diuretic-induced metabolic derangements. African-American patients have a tendency to display salt-sensitive hypertension, which is further potentiated by the presence of diabetes. Consequently, diuretics are useful in this population.

β-Blockers were shown to be particularly effective in the United Kingdom Prospective Diabetes Study (UKPDS) and the Captopril Prevention Project (CAPP) trials. These European studies involved both β-blockers and ACE inhibitors, often in combination with diuretics. Researchers in the UKPDS found that blood pressure lowering with an atenolol (Tenormin®)-based regimen was as effective as a captopril (Capoten®)-based regimen in reducing the incidence of microvascular and macrovascular diabetic complications. The CAPP study involved almost 11,000 patients who were randomized to either (1) captopril doses of up to 100 mg/day with a diuretic, if necessary, or (2) the physician's choice of either a diuretic or a β-blocker, with the opposite agent as add-on therapy, if necessary. The diabetic subgroup of 572 patients was found to have a reduction in cardiovascular end points (stroke, myocardial infarction), with a suggestion of a benefit in the ACE inhibitor/diuretic group versus the β-blocker/diuretic group. The CAPP study may have had some experimental bias because it was open label and not specifically designed to single out patients with diabetes. Additionally, these studies did not include a large cohort of minority patients easily comparable to African Americans. While the data are not conclusive in showing one agent as superior to the others, they suggest that blood pressure lowering should be the major goal, placing less importance on the type of agent used.

The Hypertension Optimal Treatment (HOT) trial showed that most cardiovascular benefit was achieved at blood pressures < 140/90 mm Hg, with the optimal pressure at 137/83 mm Hg. The study included 1,501 patients with diabetes who showed a significant cardiovascular benefit with a diastolic blood pressure of < 80 mm Hg compared to < 85 mm Hg and < 90 mm Hg. This provides possible evidence against the so-called J-curve, which states that patients with diastolic blood pressure that is too low (< 90) will have a worse cardiovascular outcome. There was no evidence of a J-curve in the < 80 mm Hg group, although the actual diastolic blood pressure in the three groups only differed by 2 mm Hg (85, 83, and 81 mm Hg). The initial goal was to divide the patients into

Table 3-4: HOPE: Key Baseline Characteristics

	Ramipril (N = 4,645)	Placebo (N = 4,652)
Mean age (years)	66	66
Female (%)	27.5	25.8
Any CAD (%)	79.5	81.4
Myocardial infarction (%)	51.9	53.4
PVD (%)	42.3	44.8
Stroke + TIA (%)	10.8	11.0
Diabetes (%)	38.9	38.0
Hypertension (%)	47.6	46.1
High cholesterol (%)	65.4	66.4

CAD = coronary artery disease, PVD = peripheral vascular disease, TIA = transient ischemic attack.

Yusuf et al, *N Engl J Med* 2000;342:145-153.

three different achieved diastolic blood pressure groups: (1) < 90 mm Hg, (2) < 85 mm Hg, and (3) < 80 mm Hg. Felodipine (Plendil®) was used in addition to either an ACE inhibitor, a diuretic, or a β-blocker to achieve goal blood pressure. More than 90% of the patients achieved a diastolic blood pressure of < 90 mm Hg with multidrug therapy, and, as a result, there were fewer cardiovascular effects than in many other hypertension trials.

The Heart Outcomes Prevention Evaluation (HOPE) trial gave a new perspective on the treatment of vascular

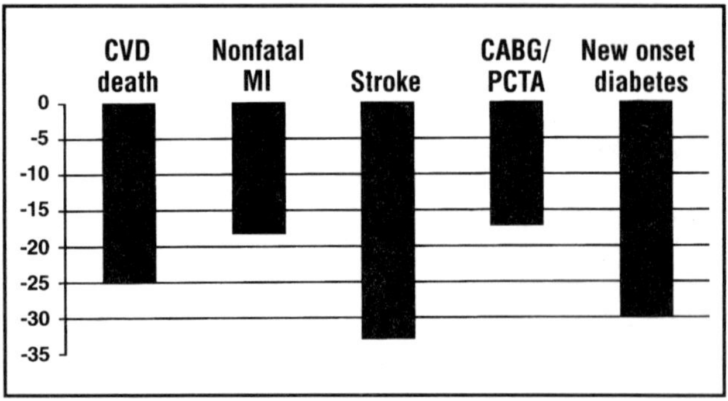

Figure 3-2: HOPE risk reduction (ACE inhibitors vs placebo). CABG = coronary artery bypass graft, CVD = cardiovascular disease, MI = myocardial infarction, PTCA = percutaneous transluminal coronary angioplasty. Source: Yusuf et al, *N Engl J Med* 2000;342:145-153.

disease. The study found that even in the absence of left ventricular dysfunction, ramipril (Altace®), an ACE inhibitor, reduced cardiovascular events in high-risk patients with or without high blood pressure. A high-risk patient was defined as one who showed evidence of cerebrovascular, coronary, or peripheral vascular disease or of diabetes with one other cardiovascular risk factor, such as hypertension, smoking, dyslipidemia, or microalbuminuria. The profile of the subjects enrolled in the HOPE trial is shown in Table 3-4. The results (illustrated in Figure 3-2) were so significant that the study was terminated early because of a 22% reduction in the primary end point, namely, the composite risk of myocardial infarction, stroke, or cardiovascular mortality. In addition, there was a 16% reduction in total mortality in the ACE-inhibitor group. The cardiovascular benefit from the ACE inhibitor, ramipril, was seen in almost all the subgroups, including those with and without diabetes or hypertension. Among the most interesting results was the reduction by about 30%

in new onset of diabetes in subjects treated with the ACE inhibitor. Vitamin E was also studied but had no impact on cardiovascular outcome or cancer incidence.

Less than 50% of the HOPE trial participants had hypertension. Those treated with ramipril, regardless of hypertension, showed a 3-mm Hg drop in systolic blood pressure and a 2-mm Hg drop in diastolic pressure. The cardiovascular benefits of ramipril were greater than expected and occurred irrespective of existing preventive therapy such as aspirin, lipid-lowering therapy, and β-blockers (Figure 3-2). Clinicians may want to consider adding an ACE inhibitor to the treatment regimen of high-risk diabetic patients and, possibly, nondiabetic patients at high risk for vascular disease (eg, smokers, hyperlipidemic patients). We have speculated that most hypertensive African-Americans may belong in a high-risk category because of their tendency to develop premature and severe cardiac disease more frequently than other populations. Chapter 6 will further examine the possible implications of the HOPE trial in the treatment of high-risk hypertensive patients, such as African Americans, even though an insignificant number of African Americans were included in the trial.

Diabetic nephropathy is a particularly significant concern for African Americans. Renal disease progression is a continuous function of blood pressure to levels of 125 to 130 mm Hg systolic and 70 to 75 mm Hg diastolic. These arterial blood pressures are associated with a significant decline in both renal disease development and renal disease progression in patients with diabetic nephropathy. Specifically, nephropathy in type 2 diabetes was shown to progress at a slower rate with intensive blood pressure control (< 140/90 mm Hg). Two recent clinical trials involving patients with type 2 diabetes found that those randomized to an ACE inhibitor or to a nondihydropyridine calcium-channel blocker had a greater reduction in proteinuria, and therefore a slower rate of renal

Table 3-5: Points to Remember About Diabetes

- In 1998, 1.5 million African Americans were known to have diabetes. This is almost 4 times the number of African Americans with diagnosed diabetes in 1968.
- About 730,000 African Americans have diabetes but do not know it.
- Among blacks aged 50 years or older, 19% of men and 28% of women have diabetes.
- Being overweight or physically inactive is a major risk factor for developing diabetes.
- Healthy lifestyles, such as eating healthy foods and getting regular exercise, are particularly important for people who are at increased risk of diabetes. Some diabetes may be prevented with weight control and regular exercise.
- African Americans have higher incidence of, and greater disability from, diabetes complications such as visual impairment, kidney failure, and need for amputation.
- If African Americans can prevent, reverse, or control their diabetes, their risk of developing complications will decrease.

National Institute of Diabetes and Digestive and Kidney Disease: *Diabetes in African Americans.* NIH Publication no. 98-3266, 1998.

disease development and progression, than those in the β-blocker group. Recent clinical trials using ARBs showed irbesartan to be effective in reducing nephropathy (IRMA-2) and significantly better than amlodipine or conventional antihypertensive agents (IDNT) in protecting renal function. In the RENAAL trial, losartan also protected against progression of nephropathy compared with conventional antihypertensive agents. In contrast to ACE inhibitors, the classes of drugs that do not reduce proteinuria—such as α-blockers, dihydropyridine calcium-channel blockers, and direct vasodilators (ie, hydralazine [Apresoline®] and minoxidil [Loniten®])—have not been shown to slow renal disease progression.

Take-home Points on Diabetic, Hypertensive Patients

- Screen all African Americans for diabetes and hypertension, since these conditions are often asymptomatic and occur frequently in this population (Table 3-5).
- Be familiar with national guidelines from the American Diabetes Association and the Joint National Committee on Prevention, Detection, Evaluation, and Treatment of High Blood Pressure on blood glucose, lipids, and blood pressure goals (Table 3-6).
- Always treat to goal blood pressure, regardless of which agents you must use to achieve this goal. Note that the clinical practice recommendations of the American Diabetes Association indicate the goal blood pressure to be 130/80 or less.
- Know the compelling indications for various antihypertensive agents, such as ACE inhibitors, for diabetic patients.
- Use simple, preferably once-daily, treatment regimens.
- Consider combination therapy, especially for patients with concomitant disease. For example, a post-myocardial infarction patient with poor systolic function should receive an ACE inhibitor and a β-blocker, if tolerated. If blood pressure is not controlled, then add a diuretic or a dihydropyridine calcium-channel blocker (Figure 3-1).
- If a patient has resistant hypertension, consider referral to a hypertension specialist certified by the American Society of Hypertension (Table 3-7).

Table 3-6: Treatment Goals for Diabetic Patients

Factors	Comments
Blood Glucose	
• Fasting blood glucose ≤ 120 • 2-hour postprandial glucose ≤ 180 • Hemoglobin A_{1C} < 7.0	Delay/prevent microvascular complications.
Lipids	
• Total cholesterol < 200 • Low-density lipoprotein cholesterol < 100 • High-density lipoprotein cholesterol ≥ 50	Levels known to avoid microvascular event rates. Triglycerides are best reduced after achieving goal blood glucose.
Blood pressure	
< 130/80 unless greater than 1 g proteinuria, then level is < 125/75	Levels known to reduce both micro- and macrovascular disease.

Modified from Gavin, *ABC Digest Urban Cardiology* 1999;6:18.

Insulin Resistance

Insulin resistance is an impaired biologic response by tissues to insulin. Insulin resistance is not the same as the insulin resistance syndrome, which was once called syndrome X but was renamed to avoid confusion with the cardiology term 'syndrome X,' which refers to chest pain without obvious coronary disease. Insulin resistance refers to impaired utilization of insulin and presents in patients as a group of related clinical and laboratory fea-

Table 3-7: Hypertension Specialists

1. The American Society of Hypertension (ASH) has created the ASH Specialist Program, which recognizes physicians with specific expertise in the management of hypertension.
2. These designated specialists accept referrals for refractory or complex hypertension cases and act as regional consultants.
3. For a list of the currently designated specialists, call ASH headquarters at (212) 696-9099 or visit the ASH Web site at www.ash-us.org.

tures, including android obesity, hypertension, dyslipidemia, glucose intolerance, and altered fibrinolysis (Table 3-8). Because of the cardiovascular and metabolic implications of insulin resistance, the term *cardiovascular dysmetabolic syndrome* was coined. Insulin resistance appears in other clinical situations, such as polycystic ovary syndrome and chronic corticosteroid treatment.

How does the clinician diagnose insulin resistance, and what is the proposed mechanism for its induced complications? One easy way to determine insulin resistance is to measure the plasma insulin level after an overnight fast. However, there are several problems with this method, including variability in results among different laboratories. In the office setting, measuring the waist-to-hip ratio, glucose level, and lipid levels provides enough data to diagnose insulin resistance. Waist-to-hip ratio is considered significant if it is > 0.95 in males and > 0.85 in females. The dyslipidemia most commonly associated with insulin resistance includes an elevated triglyceride level and a low high-density lipoprotein (HDL) cholesterol level. Based on current data, the prob-

Table 3-8: Patient Traits Associated With Insulin Resistance

Characteristics	Definition
• Impaired fasting glucose	Fasting plasma glucose 111 to 125 mg/dL 2-h glucose on OGTT of 140 to 199 mg/dL
• Impaired glucose tolerance or type 2 diabetes mellitus	Fasting plasma glucose ≥ 126 mg/dL
• Hypertriglyceridemia	Fasting plasma triglycerides ≥ 175 mg/dL
• Low HDL-C	Fasting plasma HDL < 45 mg/dL
• Centrally overweight	Body mass index > 27 kg/m^2
• Hyperuricemia or gout	
• Family history of diabetes mellitus or CAD	

CAD = coronary artery disease
HDL-C = high-density lipoprotein cholesterol
OGTT = oral glucose tolerance test

Reprinted with permission from *Geriatrics* 2000;55: 28-32, 35. *Geriatrics* is a copyrighted publication of Advanstar Communications Inc. All rights reserved.

able mechanism for developing insulin-induced and obesity-induced hypertension and dyslipidemia is illustrated in Figure 3-3. Insulin resistance has been found in blacks living in Europe as well as in those living in the United States, with one group of investigators observing that

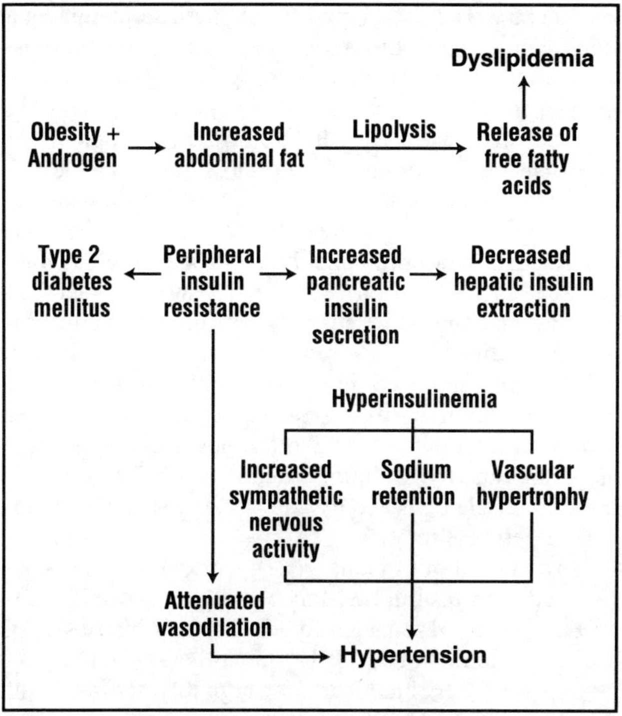

Figure 3-3: Overall scheme for the mechanism by which obesity (particularly if predominantly upper body or visceral in location) can promote diabetes, dyslipidemia, and hypertension via hyperinsulinemia. Kaplan NM: *Clinical Hypertension,* 7th ed. Philadelphia, Lippincott, Williams and Wilkins, 1998, p 78.

the resultant hyperlipidemia in blacks closely correlates with blood pressure sensitivity to sodium.

Hypertension occurs more commonly in obese individuals, partly because of insulin resistance and the associated hyperinsulinemia that occurs as a result of increased fat mass. However, nonobese patients can also have hyperinsulinemia. The data supporting hyperinsulinemia as a significant factor in the genesis of hypertension continue to accumulate. Follow-up observations of both European and American populations have found that high fasting levels of insulin were predictive of the development of hypertension. Unfortunately, no large study has definitively shown that treatment of insulin resistance will stop the development of hypertension. Importantly, the insulin sensitizer metformin and the glitazones, such as rosiglitazone and pioglitazone, have been found to lower blood pressure and should be strongly considered for insulin-resistant patients.

Metformin has been shown to lower blood pressure by blocking calcium influx into the vascular cellular bed, relaxing the arterial wall. The glitazones may act to lower blood pressure by inhibiting calcium influx into vascular smooth muscle cells and by attenuating vascular smooth muscle cell proliferation.

How should physicians treat hypertension that is associated with insulin resistance? Although insulin sensitizers may have some antihypertensive properties, they probably should not be used as monotherapy to treat hypertension. ACE inhibitors are arguably the drugs of choice, since the HOPE study showed not only a reduction in cardiovascular mortality, but also a lower incidence of new onset of diabetes in the ACE-inhibitor group. Clinicians should keep in mind that many African-American patients will require high-dose therapy when using ACE inhibitors, and it is important to use whatever combination or single drug is necessary to achieve goal blood pressure.

Dyslipidemia

Hypertensive people have a higher prevalence of hyperlipidemia than normotensive people, regardless of whether they are on therapy. Hyperlipidemia is associated with vascular endothelial dysfunction and appears to cause this dysfunction by interfering with endothelial-derived relaxing factors such as nitric oxide. Hyperlipidemia can also cause structural dysfunction of the vasculature through atherosclerosis. All hypertensive patients should be screened for lipid abnormalities and then treated aggressively with lifestyle modifications and/or pharmacologic therapy.

African Americans have lower total serum cholesterol levels than whites with a similar rate of hyperlipidemia. The Multiple Risk Factor Intervention Trial (MRFIT) showed that the relationship between total cholesterol and coronary heart disease was the same among 23,490 black men as it was among approximately 325,000 white men over an average follow-up period of 12 years. This finding contrasts with the disparity in the relationship of hypertension to cardiac disease in blacks versus whites. The first National Health and Examination Survey epidemiologic follow-up study found that African-American women did not exhibit a consistent relationship between total cholesterol levels and coronary artery disease.

African Americans tend to have a more favorable lipid profile than whites, with lower total serum cholesterol and triglyceride levels and higher concentrations of the protective HDL cholesterol. However, these findings should not be interpreted as a reason to treat African Americans with dyslipidemia less aggressively than whites. There is a significant disparity between the number of African Americans and whites involved in clinical lipid trials, and more clinical trials are needed. Until clinical trials prove otherwise, physicians should treat dyslipidemia aggressively, regardless of race.

Updates to the National Cholesterol Education Program (NCEP) are listed in Table 3-9. Table 3-10 clarifies the newly developed Framingham risk assessment. When treating hypertensive patients with dyslipidemia, physicians should know that hyperlipidemia is not a rea-

Table 3-9: New Features of ATP III

Focus on multiple risk factors.

Persons with diabetes without coronary heart disease (CHD) (most of whom have multiple risk factors) are raised to the risk level of CHD risk equivalent, as are individuals with multiple (2+) risk factors and a 10-year risk of a heart attack > 20%. Framingham risk scoring is used to identify patients with multiple (2+) risk factors who need more intensive treatment. In addition, persons with multiple metabolic risk factors (metabolic syndrome) are identified as candidates for intensified therapeutic lifestyle changes (TLC).

A complete lipoprotein profile is recommended as the first test to measure cholesterol.

ATP III advises healthy adults to have a fasting lipoprotein profile once every 5 years, beginning at age 20. A complete lipoprotein profile is preferred to the previous recommendation of measuring total cholesterol and high-density lipoprotein (HDL) cholesterol.

Lipids and lipoproteins are reclassified.

A low-density lipoprotein (LDL) cholesterol level of < 100 mg/dL is classified as 'optimal,' and the categorical low HDL cholesterol value is raised to < 40 mg/dL, an increase from the previous level of < 35 mg/dL. In addition, triglycerides < 150 mg/dL are considered normal (compared to < 200 mg/dL in ATP II), and greater attention is given to moderate elevations.

son to withhold diuretics and β-blockers in the presence of compelling indications, especially since many African Americans require diuretics for blood pressure control. The use of β-blockers and diuretics has declined significantly in the past 20 years, partly because of cli-

New set of therapeutic lifestyle changes that are more powerful at lowering cholesterol.

ATP III recommends a more intense and effective eating plan than previously used. The TLC diet allows up to 35% of daily calories from total fat for some people, provided that most consist of unsaturated fat, which does not raise cholesterol levels. (A lower carbohydrate intake may be needed by some patients with high triglycerides and/or a low HDL to keep their triglycerides or HDL levels from worsening.) In the TLC diet, plant stanols/sterols (found in cholesterol-lowering margarines) and soluble fiber may be added to the diet to further lower LDL cholesterol. A key part of TLC is weight control and physical activity; both are intensified in order to improve various heart disease risk factors.

Increased attention to triglycerides after the LDL goal is reached.

ATP III recommends treatment beyond LDL lowering for persons who have triglycerides ≥ 200 mg/dL and/or low HDL level.

ATP III = Third Report of the National Cholesterol Education Program Expert Panel on Detection, Evaluation, and Treatment of High Blood Cholesterol in Adults (Adult Treatment Panel III)

New features of ATP III. *Heartmemo* Spring 2002.

nicians' concern about a potentially negative effect of these two classes on plasma lipids and glucose. This effect has not been shown to negate the positive effect that diuretics and β-blockers have on coronary disease. In a recent study, β-blockers and diuretics did not signifi-

Table 3-10: Framingham Point Scores Estimate of 10-Year Risk for Men

Age, years	Points
20-34	-9
35-39	-4
40-44	0
45-49	3
50-54	6
55-59	8
60-64	10
65-69	11
70-74	12
75-79	13

Total Cholesterol, mg/dL	Points Age 20-39 y	Age 40-49 y	Age 50-59 y	Age 60-69 y	Age 70-79 y
< 160	0	0	0	0	0
160-199	4	3	2	1	0
200-239	7	5	3	1	0
240-279	9	6	4	2	1
≥ 280	11	8	5	3	1

	Points Age 20-39 y	Age 40-49 y	Age 50-59 y	Age 60-69 y	Age 70-79 y
Nonsmoker	0	0	0	0	0
Smoker	8	5	3	1	1

HDL-C, mg/dL	Points
≥ 60	-1
50-59	0
40-49	1
< 40	2

Systolic BP, mm Hg	If Untreated	If Treated
< 120	0	0
120-129	0	1
130-139	1	2
140-159	1	2
≥ 160	2	3

Point Total	10-Year Risk (%)
< 0	< 1
0	1
1	1
2	1
3	1
4	1
5	2
6	2
7	3
8	4
9	5
10	6
11	8
12	10
13	12
14	16
15	20
16	25
≥ 17	≥ 30

(continued on next page)

Table 3-10: Framingham Point Scores Estimate of 10-Year Risk for Women *(continued)*

Age, years	Points
20-34	-7
35-39	-3
40-44	0
45-49	3
50-54	6
55-59	8
60-64	10
65-69	12
70-74	14
75-79	16

Total Cholesterol, mg/dL	Points Age 20-39 y	Age 40-49 y	Age 50-59 y	Age 60-69 y	Age 70-79 y
< 160	0	0	0	0	0
160-199	4	3	2	1	1
200-239	8	6	4	2	1
240-279	11	8	5	3	2
≥ 280	13	10	7	4	2

	Points Age 20-39 y	Age 40-49 y	Age 50-59 y	Age 60-69 y	Age 70-79 y
Nonsmoker	0	0	0	0	0
Smoker	9	7	4	2	1

HDL-C, mg/dL	Points
≥ 60	-1
50-59	0
40-49	1
< 40	2

Systolic BP, mm Hg	If Untreated	If Treated
< 120	0	0
120-129	1	3
130-139	2	4
140-159	3	5
≥ 160	4	6

Point Total	10-Year Risk (%)
< 9	< 1
9	1
10	1
11	1
12	1
13	2
14	2
15	3
16	4
17	5
18	6
19	8
20	11
21	14
22	17
23	22
24	27
≥ 25	≥ 30

cantly alter the overall lipid profile over a 1-year period. However, not all diuretics affect lipids in the same way. Potassium-sparing diuretics have little, if any, effect on lipids compared to thiazide and loop diuretics. β-blockers without intrinsic sympathetic activity tend to raise triglycerides, lower HDL cholesterol, and variably affect total serum cholesterol. Conversely, β-blockers with intrinsic sympathetic activity and those with α-blocking properties, such as labetalol (Normodyne®, Trandate®) and carvedilol (Coreg®), produce no appreciable effects on lipid levels (Table 3-11).

Do lipid-lowering agents interfere with antihypertensive therapy? There are five classes of lipid-lowering agents: bile acid sequestrates, nicotinic acid, statins, fibric acid derivatives, and probucol (no longer available in the United States). Bile acid sequestrates often interfere with antihypertensive drug absorption. One study showed a beneficial effect of an ACE inhibitor and statin combination, resulting in greater reduction in blood pressure than when the ACE inhibitor was used alone. Nicotinic acid may increase the decline in blood pressure when given in combination with direct vasodilators such as minoxidil or hydralazine.

Renal failure patients have a higher risk of myopathy when given fibric acid derivatives (eg, gemfibrozil [Lopid®]) compared with the normal population. The risk of myopathy also increases in renal failure patients who take statins. Fortunately, many patients can usually be treated with statins, which are highly effective and usually well tolerated. In addition, preliminary reports indicate that statins may lower blood pressure by improving the endothelial function of blood vessels.

Because patients' responses vary, regular monitoring of lipid levels is important. Most clinical trials have looked at lowering low-density lipoprotein (LDL) cholesterol, and most authors seem to agree that this should be the first priority in lipid therapy.

Table 3-11: Effect of Antihypertensive Agents on Serum Lipids

Agent	Effect on Serum Lipids
• Calcium antagonists	No significant change
• Angiotensin-converting enzyme inhibitors	No significant change
• Angiotensin-receptor blockers	No significant change
• Hydralazine	No significant change
• Minoxidil	No significant change
• Potassium-sparing diuretics	No significant change
• Reserpine	No significant change
• Thiazide diuretics at higher doses (≥ 25 mg)	Increase LDL, total cholesterol but no effect on HDL cholesterol; increase triglycerides
• Loop diuretics	Same as thiazide diuretics except for lower HDL cholesterol levels
• α-receptor blockers	Mild decrease in total cholesterol and LDL cholesterol
• Central α-agonists	Mild decrease in total cholesterol and LDL cholesterol
• β-blockers without intrinsic sympathomimetic activity	Reduce HDL; increase triglycerides
• β-blockers with α-blocking properties	No significant change

Table 3-12: The Effects of Weight Loss on the Incidence of Hypertension in Trials of Lifestyle Modifications

Trial	Number of Patients	Duration (Years)
Primary Prevention of Hypertension (1989)	201	5
Hypertension Prevention Trial (1990)	252	3
Trials of Hypertension Prevention (TOHP)		
I (TOHP 1992)	565	1.5
II (TOHP 1997)	595	4

Kaplan NM: *Clinical Hypertension,* 7th ed. Philadelphia, Lippincott, Williams and Wilkins, 1998, p 174.

Diet

A short ride through almost any large African-American neighborhood will illustrate the problem of poor dietary habits in this population. Fast-food businesses are everywhere, and many supermarkets have small inventories of low-sodium, low-fat products. Chapter 8 examines how these problems can be addressed in a community-oriented way, but this section focuses on how compliance with dietary restrictions can lower blood pressure.

When discussing dietary habits with patients, it is important to focus on realistic goals that can be reached and sustained, rather than far-reaching goals that usually bring only temporary success. Therefore, any dietary

Weight Loss (kg)	Reduction of Incidence %
2.7	54
1.6	23
3.9	51
1.9	21

modification plan should always start with urging patients to reduce the portions of food they eat. Despite the availability of food labeling, many Americans still consume more calories, sodium, fat, and cholesterol than needed. If a specific diet is necessary, the Dietary Approaches to Stop Hypertension (DASH) diet outlined in JNC 7 should be considered. This diet was shown to be more effective in lowering systolic and diastolic blood pressure in hypertensive African Americans than in hypertensive whites. The DASH study found that a diet high in fruits, vegetables, and low-fat dairy products reduced blood pressure more significantly than one only rich in vegetables and fruits (control diet).

Dietary modifications can lower blood pressure, but more studies are needed to determine whether lowering blood pressure through diet has a similar impact on cardiovascular morbidity and mortality when compared to therapy with antihypertensive agents (Table 3-12). At present, clinicians should recommend dietary changes to lower sodium and reduce weight in selected hypertensive patients. The lifestyle modifications listed in Table 6-1, Chapter 6, are likely to be effective, particularly in African Americans, and are less expensive than drug therapy alone.

Dietary elements such as magnesium, caffeine, protein, and garlic may prove to have an impact on blood pressure. Magnesium has received some attention because of its efficacy in treating pregnant women with eclampsia. However, there are not enough convincing data to recommend increasing magnesium intake to lower blood pressure. Caffeine raises blood pressure on an acute, short-term basis, and tolerance develops very quickly. Garlic has not yet been shown to reduce blood pressure in multiple, large clinical trials (see Chapter 6).

Changing a patient's dietary habits often requires behavior modification techniques that clinicians may find difficult to implement in the office setting. Offering patients simple advice, such as cutting portions in half and eating meals without bread and butter, is recommended.

In summary, all hypertensive patients should be educated on nutrition, and physicians need to be better trained in dietary counseling because many insurance plans will not allow a referral to a registered dietitian. Additionally, physicians should note that sustained dietary habit changes and weight loss are goals that can only be met with a combination of dietary counseling, exercise, and behavior modifications. Unfortunately, in many African-American communities, exercise facilities and healthy eating facilities (ie, those offering low-fat, well-balanced meals) are scarce, so reducing caloric intake is particularly important.

Sodium Restriction

During the 1940s, sodium restriction and other essentially unproven therapies were the only hypertension treatments offered. By the 1950s, thiazide diuretics were available as antihypertensive therapy. Recently, some researchers have advanced the idea that sodium restriction may not necessarily help in reducing hypertension. While most Western diets contain many times the recommended daily adult sodium requirements, only a portion of the population develops hypertension, likely because sodium-sensitive people have a defect in sodium excretion not found in the normotensive population.

How should the clinician advise patients about sodium restriction, especially since a 'salt controversy' is beginning to emerge? First, clinicians should not forget that restricting sodium in the very old is beneficial, especially since sodium sensitivity increases with age. Second, even proponents of a low-sodium diet agree that more research is needed to determine sodium's effect on blood pressure. Overall, however, the majority of clinicians and researchers support dietary sodium restriction. For the present, clinicians should review the NIH's JNC 7 report, which endorses the DASH diet. An analysis of previous diet studies has correlated a 5.8-mm Hg reduction in systolic pressure with a 100 mmol/day urinary sodium reduction.

Although controversy exists among nutritional experts about which diet is best, certain key principles should be kept in mind. Any diet aimed toward good cardiovascular health promotes a large intake of fruits and vegetables, as noted in the DASH diet (Table 3-13) and the American Heart Association's diet for reducing cholesterol in higher-risk patients, previously called the Step II diet (Table 3-14). Fruits and vegetables are good sources of fiber, starch, vitamins, and minerals and are generally low in sodium. Frying and breading foods should be avoided; baking, broiling, microwaving, and roasting are better. Very low-calorie diets (500 to 800 calories/day) are usually ineffective

Table 3-13: The DASH Diet

Food Group	Daily Servings	Serving Sizes
Grains and grain products	7-8	1 slice bread 1/2 c (0.12 L) dry cereal 1/2 c (0.12 L) cooked rice, pasta, or cereal
Vegetables	4-5	1 c (0.24 L) raw, leafy vegetables 1/2 c (0.12 L) cooked vegetables 6 oz (180 mL) vegetable juice
Fruits	4-5	6 oz (180 mL) fruit juice 1 medium fruit 1/4 c (0.06 L) dried fruit 1/2 c (0.06 L) fresh, frozen, or canned fruit
Low-fat or nonfat dairy foods	2-3	8 oz (240 mL) milk 1 c (0.24 L) yogurt 1.5 oz (45 g) cheese
Meats, poultry, and fish	≤ 2	3 oz (84 g) cooked meats, poultry, or fish
Nuts, seeds, and legumes	4-5/wk	1.5 oz (42 g) or 1/3 c (0.08 L) nuts 0.5 oz (14 g) or 2 tbsp (3 mL) seeds 1/2 c (0.12 L) cooked legumes

National Heart, Lung, and Blood Institute: *JNC 7 Express: The Seventh Report of the Joint National Committee on Prevention, Detection, Evaluation, and Treatment of High Blood Pressure.*

Examples and Notes	**Significance to the DASH Diet Pattern**
Whole wheat bread, English muffin, pita bread, bagel, cereals, grits, oatmeal	Major sources of energy and fiber
Tomatoes, potatoes, carrots, peas, squash, broccoli, turnip greens, collards, kale, spinach, artichokes, beans, sweet potatoes	Rich sources of potassium, magnesium, and fiber
Apricots, bananas, dates, grapes, oranges, orange juice, mangoes, melons, peaches, pineapples, prunes, raisins, strawberries, tangerines	Important sources of potassium, magnesium, and fiber
Skim or 1% milk, skim or low-fat buttermilk, nonfat or low-fat yogurt, mozzarella cheese, part-skim mozzarella cheese, nonfat cheese	Major sources of calcium and protein
Select only lean meats; trim away visible fats; broil instead of frying; remove skin from poultry	Rich sources of protein and magnesium
Almonds, filberts, mixed nuts, peanuts, walnuts, sunflower seeds, kidney beans, lentils	Rich sources of energy, magnesium, potassium, protein, and fiber

Rockville, MD, US Department of Health and Human Services; May 2003. NIH Publication no. 03-5233.

Table 3-14: AHA Diet for Lowering the Risk of Heart Disease*

- Saturated fat < 7% of total calories
- Total fat < 30% of total calories
- Cholesterol < 200 mg/day
- Total calories to achieve and maintain ideal body weight

* Replaces Step II diet.

AHA = American Heart Association.

Available from http://www.americanheart.org.

for achieving long-term weight loss for most patients. Clinicians should provide patients with tangible visual aids, such as food product labels, as references.

Several studies have found that mild sodium restriction can significantly enhance the efficacy of almost all antihypertensive agents. Conversely, high sodium intake seems to have a significant adverse effect on the efficacy of antihypertensive agents, especially ACE inhibitors.

In summary, it is practical to recommend restricting sodium intake to 2 to 4 g per day, best achieved by encouraging patients to read food labels and eliminate added salt in food preparation. Potassium supplements were also found to have a significant positive impact on blood pressure, with several studies showing a 4.4-mm Hg drop in systolic pressure when supplements of 50 to 120 mEq per day were used. Patients can be advised to restrict sodium, to eat more potassium-rich foods such as bananas, and to consider taking 1.5 g of elemental calcium daily, which seems to reduce blood pressure slightly in some patients and decrease the risk of osteoporosis.

Specific issues concerning African Americans, hypertension, and salt consumption should be addressed. African Americans of lower socioeconomic status tend to consume more sodium than those of higher socioeconomic status, so the clinician must be aware of subgroups within the African-American community that may need different approaches to hypertension. A larger portion of hypertensive African Americans are salt sensitive compared to their white hypertensive counterparts, and, most importantly, salt-sensitive hypertensive patients tend to have higher blood pressure medication requirements. This is particularly relevant for ACE inhibitors and β-blockers. However, in a study by Weir et al, the antihypertensive efficiency of valsartan (Diovan®), an angiotensin-receptor inhibitor, was not significantly attenuated by a high-salt (200 mEq/day) diet in hypertensive African Americans. In most salt-sensitive patients, calcium antagonists will have a significant antihypertensive effect, but even this class of drugs will be partially affected by a high-sodium diet.

Take-home Points on Sodium

The following points were discussed at the National Heart, Lung, and Blood Institute (NHLBI) Workshop on Sodium and Hypertension held in 1999:

- Nearly 80% of the salt consumed in the American diet comes from processed foods. (See Table 3-15 for a list of low-salt, high-potassium natural foods.)
- Salt sensitivity increases with age.
- Overweight elderly patients may receive greater benefit from sodium restriction.
- Persons at high risk for hypertension (especially blacks) exhibit better responses to sodium reduction.
- Minerals other than sodium, such as calcium, magnesium, and potassium, also affect blood pressure.
- Studies of single nutrients may not be relevant because foods contain multiple nutrients.
- Studies reporting the adverse effects of a low-sodium diet either have not been replicated or contain unanswered methodologic problems.

Table 3-15: Low-Salt, High-Potassium Foods

Food	Serving Size	Potassium* (mg)	Sodium** (mg)
Apricots	3 medium	281	1
Apricots (dried)	8 halves	490	13
Asparagus	6 spears	278	2
Avocado	1/2 medium	604	4
Banana	1 medium	569	1
Beans (white, cooked)	1/2 cup	416	7
Beans (green)	1 cup	189	5
Broccoli	1 stalk	267	10
Cantaloupe	1/4 medium	251	12
Carrots	2 small	341	47
Dates	10 medium	648	1
Grapefruit	1/2 medium	135	1
Mushrooms	4 large	414	15
Orange	1 medium	311	2
Orange juice	1 cup	496	3
Peach	1 medium	202	1
Peanuts (plain)	2 1/2 oz	740	2
Potato	1 medium	504	4
Prunes (dried)	8 large	940	11
Raisins	1/4 medium	271	10
Spinach	1/2 cup	291	45
Squash (acorn)	1/2 baked	749	2
Sunflower seeds	3 1/2 oz	920	30
Sweet potato	1 small	367	15
Tomato	1 small	244	3
Watermelon	1 slice (6 1/2 in)	600	6

* 1,000 mg = 25.6 mmol

** 1,000 mg = 44 mmol

Moser M: *Clinical Management of Hypertension.* Caddo (OK): Professional Communications, Inc, 1996, p 30. Reprinted with permission.

Cigarette Smoking, Alcohol, and Substance Abuse

Cigarette Smoking

Cigarette smoking should be avoided, and all patients who smoke should be advised to quit. In the past, it was thought that tolerance to the acute pressure effect of nicotine developed quickly and therefore that tobacco use did not significantly affect blood pressure. It was also thought that because chronic smokers often weigh less than nonsmokers, they are not at as much risk for hypertension resulting from excess weight. However, it is now recognized that smoking does increase blood pressure, but the effect only lasts about 30 minutes after each cigarette, and tolerance to nicotine's blood pressure effect does not develop. For the clinician, this means that when blood pressure is measured in a smoke-free environment, the nicotine-induced rise in pressure may be missed.

Smoking cessation is not an easy task for many patients and is probably best approached with multiple methods, such as a nicotine patch (Habitrol®, NicoDerm CQ®, Nicotrol®, ProStep®) combined with smoking cessation classes. Smokeless tobacco and cigars are not recommended as substitutes to cigarette smoking because they can increase blood pressure, are not usually well tolerated, and present other health risks. Various pharmacologic agents have been tried for smoking cessation, with the antidepressant bupropion receiving the most attention.

Combination therapy, including smoking cessation classes and pharmacologic therapy (Table 3-16), is usually needed to successfully stop smoking. If a patient is unable to quit, there is some indication that vigorous exercise may mitigate the cardiovascular risk of smoking.

Take-home Points for Cigarette Smoking and Hypertension

- Any tobacco use increases the risk of cardiovascular disease.

Table 3-16: Smoking Cessation Agents

Brand	Strength(s)
Transdermal	
Habitrol® (active ingredient: nicotine)	21 mg/24 h 14 mg/24 h 7 mg/24 h
NicoDerm CQ® (active ingredient: nicotine)	OTC: 21 mg/24 h 14 mg/24 h 7 mg/24 h
Nicotrol Transdermal® (active ingredient: nicotine)	OTC: 15 mg/16 h

Modified from Clinical Practice Guideline, No. 18, AHCPR Publication No. 96-0692, April 1996; relevant product labeling; and *Monthly Prescribing Reference.* New York, Prescribing Reference, Inc, a division of Haymarket Media, October 2002, p 262.

Dose	Comments
One 21 mg/24 h patch daily for 4-8 wk, then one 14 mg/24 h patch for 2-4 wk, then one 7 mg/24 h patch daily for 2-4 wk; then discontinue.	Apply to clean, dry, nonhairy site on trunk or upper outer arm. Rotate sites.
Usual: One 21 mg/24 h patch daily for 4-8 wk, then one 14 mg/24 h patch for 2 wk, then one 7 mg/ 24 h patch for 2 wk; then discontinue. *Low-dose regimen:* One 14 mg/24 h patch daily for 6 wk, then one 7 mg/24 h patch daily for 2 wk; then discontinue.	Apply to clean, dry, nonhairy site on trunk or upper outer arm. Rotate sites. Remove after 16-24 h.
One patch worn for 16 h daily for 6 wk; then discontinue.	Apply to clean, dry, nonhairy site on hip or upper outer arm. Remove at bedtime. Rotate sites. Not for use in light smokers.

(continued on next page)

Table 3-16: Smoking Cessation Agents *(continued)*

Brand	Strength(s)
Chewing Gum	
Nicorette® (active ingredient: nicotine)	OTC: 2 mg 4 mg
Nasal Spray	
Nicotrol NS® (active ingredient: nicotine)	0.5-mg spray (aqueous nasal spray)
Inhaler	
Nicotrol Inhaler® (active ingredient: nicotine)	10 mg/cartridge (4 mg delivered)
Oral Dosage Form	
Zyban® (active ingredient: bupropion)	150-mg sustained-released tablets

Dose	Comments
Chew one piece every 1-2 h (at least 9/day) for 6 wk, then one piece every 2-4 h for 3 wk, then one piece every 4-8 h for 3 wk; then discontinue.	Avoid food and acidic drinks for 15 min before and during chewing. Use 4 mg strength for highly nicotine-dependent patients, or if failed with 2 mg.
Initial: 1-2 doses/h; may stop abruptly if needed. Max 5 doses/h, 40 doses/d. Max 3 months treatment. 2 sprays is one dose (one spray/nostril).	Do not sniff, swallow, or inhale spray. Nasal vasoconstrictors may delay absorption.
Use at least 6 and up to 16 cartridges/day for up to 12 wk, then (if needed) reduce gradually over 12 more wk; then discontinue. Max 6 months treatment.	20 minutes of active puffing releases 4 mg of nicotine (about 2 mg absorbed, equivalent to about 2 cigarettes).
Patients ≥ 18 y: 150 mg once daily for 3 d, then 150 mg twice daily (at least 8 h apart); max 150 mg twice daily for 7-12 wk. Patients < 18 y: not recommended (insufficient data). Reduce dose in renal or hepatic impairment.	May be used with nicotine replacement, but stop smoking within 1-2 wk of starting Zyban®. Do not crush, chew, or divide tablets. Avoid bedtime dosing. Do not use with other forms of bupropion.

- Smoking a cigarette acutely raises blood pressure within 15 to 30 minutes, and nicotine tolerance does not develop; thus, smoking will consistently elevate blood pressure, even in chronic smokers.
- Smoking cessation can produce cardiovascular benefits within a year for all age groups.
- Health practitioners must tell patients to quit smoking.
- Nicotine patches do not appear to increase blood pressure.
- Physicians should anticipate weight gain in patients who quit smoking and should provide dietary and exercise advice in advance.
- Practitioners should not delay antihypertensive therapy because they think smoking is contributing to high blood pressure. Simply ask the patient to wait 45 to 60 minutes after smoking before checking blood pressure. If the blood pressure is still elevated, proceed with antihypertensive therapy.

Alcohol Abuse

Alcohol consumption can have a positive impact on cardiovascular disease. When consumed in quantities of 1 or 2 oz per day, alcohol may lower the risk of cardiovascular morbidity and mortality. However, heavy alcohol use—defined as consuming more than 2 oz per day—raises blood pressure by producing an acute pressure response mediated by the sympathetic nervous system. Importantly, alcohol consumption does not affect everyone in the same way, especially with regard to body mass and gender. In some patients, especially thin women, small amounts of alcohol may produce a significant pressure response. Clinicians should not, then, recommend that all patients consume alcohol to lower cardiac risk.

A study published in 1977 on alcohol consumption and hypertension in blacks showed some interesting findings. The Kaiser-Permanente Multiphasic Health Examination Study (1964-1968), which included more than 12,000 black subjects, found a positive relationship between the level of blood pressure and quantity of alcohol consumed. However, in black men and women, this association between blood pressure and alcohol was not as strong as in their white counterparts. The consumption of three or more drinks per day was found to produce a significantly higher blood pressure than that found in nondrinking subjects. Consistent with the NIH's JNC 7 report on hypertension, a beneficial effect was found with the consumption of two drinks per day in black and white women. Even though the relationship between alcohol consumption and blood pressure may not be as strong in blacks as in whites, it would be prudent to follow the JNC 7 report recommendations for alcohol use. It should also be noted that a subset of patients will show complete resolution of their hypertension through alcohol abstinence, so any patient with high blood pressure should consider discontinuing alcohol consumption.

Take-home Points on Alcohol Consumption

- Excess alcohol intake (> 3 drinks per day) can raise blood pressure, cause resistance to antihypertensive therapy, and serve as a risk factor for stroke.
- Alcohol intake for men should be limited to 1 oz (30 mL) of ethanol per day (eg, 24 oz [720 mL] of beer, 10 oz [300 mL] of wine, or 2 oz [960 mL] of 100-proof whiskey). Alcohol intake should be limited to 0.5 oz (15 mL) per day for women and lighter-weight men.
- African Americans should follow the same guidelines for alcohol intake (noted above) as whites, despite data showing that blacks do not exhibit a strong relationship between alcohol consumption and blood pressure.
- Referral to an addiction specialist should be considered for alcoholic patients, since alcohol withdrawal can lead to high blood pressure and cardiac arrhythmias.

Substance Abuse

Cocaine is a potent sympathomimetic substance that is used medicinally in its hydrochloride salt form and as a recreational drug in its salt form, or in its more lipophilic 'freebase' (crack cocaine) form. Unfortunately, cocaine use has reached epidemic proportions, especially in low-income areas of large cities. Cocaine abuse can lead to a variety of medical complications, most of which are cardiovascular, such as stroke and myocardial infarction.

Cocaine produces its pharmacologic effects primarily through two physiologic actions: (1) it is a potent sympathomimetic, and (2) it is a sodium-channel blocker with various effects on myocardial functions. Most recreational users take small doses (1 to 3 mg/kg), which predominantly produce adrenergic effects. At higher doses, especially in overdose situations, depressant effects often affect sodium channels as well as cardiac conduction and function. Cocaine stimulates catecholamine release and then blocks the reuptake of these substances. The resulting increase in catecholamines acts to raise blood pressure and heart rate. Cocaine also acts as a similar agonist with serotonin and dopamine. In addition to its effects on the neurohumoral system, cocaine can act as a vasoconstrictor by increasing release of endothelin-1, a potent vasoconstrictor released from endothelial cells, while decreasing production of local nitrous oxide, a vasodilator.

Cocaine can be snorted, smoked, or injected intravenously; the route of administration can significantly affect its absorption and length of action. It is often abused in conjunction with alcohol, which can have a hypertensive effect in and of itself in some patients. An unfortunate consequence is that alcohol and cocaine together can result in a metabolite that has longer duration than cocaine alone. While most clinicians clearly understand that cocaine has an acute hypertensive effect and can lead to potentially lethal cardiac arrhythmias, many do not know that it may induce chronic hypertension and target organ damage. In fact, a major cause of stroke in young people is cocaine abuse. Cocaine use has also been associated with left ventricular hypertrophy on echocardiogram, despite a normal resting blood pressure. African-American cocaine users seem especially prone to this problem. Therefore, it is possible that repeated intermittent cocaine use may lead to end-organ damage even if chronic hypertension is not clearly documented.

The relationship between cocaine and chronic hypertension has not been clearly established, with at least two clinical trials showing no evidence of cocaine-induced chronic hypertension. One theory is that we do not find a relationship because cocaine inhibits a baroreceptor-mediated increase in blood pressure and that a person can quickly develop a tolerance to the chronotropic effects of cocaine. Despite these research findings, the presence of left ventricular hypertrophy and renal vascular changes in some cocaine users provides circumstantial evidence for cocaine-induced sustained hypertension. In practical terms, physicians should make detoxification from narcotics their first priority, since substance abuse will make treatment of hypertension more difficult. Treatment of cocaine addiction is a complex process, often requiring referral to a specialized counselor.

Use of other drugs, such as marijuana or tetrahydrocannabinol (THC) in moderate amounts, increases heart rate but usually lowers blood pressure. Heroin and other intravenously injected drugs can lead to renal failure, which raises blood pressure. Amphetamines have an effect similar to cocaine in terms of the cardiovascular system. Physicians should note that many over-the-counter cold and diet preparations contain amphetamine-like substances that can also raise blood pressure.

Take-home Points for Nonalcoholic Substance Abuse

- Illicit drug use should be suspected in cases of resistant hypertension.
- Adolescents and young adults are at especially high risk for drug abuse.
- Many substance abusers have underlying mental illness, which must be treated appropriately.

- Many addicts abuse multiple drugs, and the abuse of over-the-counter drugs should also be considered during evaluation.
- Based on available data, hypertension induced by illicit drugs is probably best treated by α-β-blockers (eg, labetalol), nitroglycerin, and calcium-channel blockers. Paradoxically, β-blockers may raise blood pressure in substance abusers. Direct vasodilators such as nitroprusside (Nitropress®) may worsen tachycardia.

Psychosocial and Socioeconomic Factors

For researchers in hypertension, the effects of psychosocial and socioeconomic issues on high blood pressure have always been a topic for discussion. This is particularly true regarding African Americans, who have traditionally been the targets of racism and economic discrimination. The debate continues: are African Americans genetically different from whites, or do socioeconomic issues play a major role in the higher prevalence of hypertension? The likely answer is that both play a part, but conclusive research is needed.

The theory that psychosocial issues cause hypertension is difficult to prove. Circumstantial evidence indicates a relationship between high blood pressure and psychosocial factors. One group of authors published a study showing that darker skin is directly proportional to the amount of stress in many black patients, and this stress probably contributes to high blood pressure. To complicate matters further, there have been internal struggles in the African-American community between light-skinned and darker-skinned people. In fact, very dark African Americans often have major difficulties climbing the socioeconomic ladder because of racism and other barriers within their community.

Socioeconomic factors can also have a major impact on hypertension treatment, particularly when it comes to choosing antihypertensive medications. African Americans tend to have higher unemployment rates, and many have no health insurance. As a result, African Americans in lower socioeconomic groups, particularly those who are asymptomatic, may not obtain hypertension treatment or blood pressure screening. Unemployment is also a major source of stress on individuals and their families, increasing the potential risk of hypertension. It is difficult to quantify the impact that low socioeconomic status has on hypertension because 90% to 95% of essential hypertension has no specific cause and is probably multifactorial in origin.

Further circumstantial evidence of the effects of environment on hypertension is noted in a study of a tribe in Kenya who lived in a rural area and showed a relatively low prevalence of hypertension. Subsequently, the tribe relocated to Nairobi, a large city, and the average blood pressure level increased substantially. After some political unrest in Nairobi, the tribe returned to the countryside, and the average blood pressure dropped to previous levels. Although a number of different factors could account for the differences in blood pressure, this observation is a good indication of the effect the environment has on hypertension.

Numerous books and articles in the popular press have suggested that stress and illness are closely linked. Some research has indicated that stress has a negative effect on the immune system, central nervous system, and cardiovascular system. Just as importantly, the research also indicated that having a positive attitude, such as strong religious faith, can significantly reduce stress and have a positive effect on health.

Finally, cultural competence (sensitivity) is an important issue in health care, not only for African Americans, but also for African-American physicians. Cultural competence is the physician's ability to understand the culture of the population he or she serves, so that cultural differences do not act as barriers to good health care.

Religion and Medicine

The church has always had a significant influence on the African-American community. Many community activists have advocated centering health education for laymen in community churches. In one study, most patients stated they want their physicians to include spiritual issues when discussing medical care, but few doctors actually do. Patients are especially likely to consider faith and spirituality important during severe illnesses.

Can religion have a positive effect on blood pressure? Evidence exists showing that people who consider themselves to be religious have lower blood pressure and lower hypertension-related morbidity and mortality. The improved morbidity and mortality were once believed to be attributable to religious persons following healthier lifestyles. But one study found that smokers who consider themselves 'not religious' were seven times more likely to have abnormally high diastolic blood pressure than 'religious' smokers. Furthermore, smokers who rarely attended church were found to be four times more likely to have an abnormally high diastolic blood pressure than regular churchgoers.

Selected Readings

Alderman MH, Madhavan S, Cohen H, et al: Low urinary sodium is associated with greater risk of myocardial infarction among treated hypertensive men. *Hypertension* 1995;25:1144-1152.

Ambre JJ, Belknap SM, Nelson J, et al: Acute tolerance to cocaine in humans. *Clin Pharmacol Ther* 1988;44:1-8.

American Diabetes Association: Treatment of hypertension in adults with diabetes. *Diabetes Care* 2003;26(suppl):S80-S82.

Aronne L: Obesity. *Med Clin North Am* 1998;82:161-181.

Bakris GL. Microalbuminuria: prognostic implications. *Curr Opin Nephrol Hypertens* 1996;5:219-223.

Bakris GL: Progression of diabetic nephropathy: a focus on arterial pressure level and methods of reduction. *Diabetes Res Clin Pract* 1998;39(suppl):S35-S42.

Bakris GL, Copley JB, Vicknair N, et al: Calcium channel blockers versus other antihypertensive therapies on progression of NIDDM associated nephropathy. *Kidney Int* 1996;50:1641-1650.

Bakris GL, Mangrum A, Copley JB, et al: Effect of calcium channel or β-blockade on the progression of diabetic nephropathy in African Americans. *Hypertension* 1997;29:744-750.

Billman GE: Mechanisms responsible for the cardiotoxic effects of cocaine. *FASEB J* 1990;4:2469-2475.

Brecklin CS, Bauman JL: Cardiovascular effects of cocaine: focus on hypertension. *J Clin Hypertens* 1999;1:212-217.

Buchanan TA, Meehan WP, Jeng YY, et al: Blood pressure lowering by pioglitazone. Evidence for a direct vascular effect. *J Clin Invest* 1995;96:354-360.

Clinical guidelines on the identification, evaluation, and treatment of overweight and obesity in adults—The Evidence Report. National Institutes of Health. *Obes Res* 1998;6(suppl 2):51S-209S.

Coleman LT: Obesity as a risk factor for cardiovascular disease. *ABC Digest Urban Cardiol* 1999;6:23-28.

Consensus development conference on insulin resistance. November 5-6,1997. American Diabetes Association. *Diabetes Care* 1998;21:310-314.

Corrigan S, Raczynski J, Swencionis C, et al: Weight reduction in the prevention and treatment of hypertension: a review of representative clinical trials. *Am J Health Promot* 1991;5:208-214.

Croft JB, Strogatz DS, Keenan NL, et al: The independent effects of obesity and body fat distribution on blood pressure in black adults: the Pitt County Study. *Int J Obes Relat Metab Disord* 1993;17:391-397.

Cruickshank JM: J curve in antihypertensive therapy—does it exist? A personal point of view. *Cardiovasc Drugs Ther* 1994;8:757-760.

Curd JD, Pressel SL, Cutler JA, et al: Effect of diuretic-based antihypertensive treatment on cardiovascular disease risk in older diabetic patients with isolated systolic hypertension. Systolic Hypertension in the Elderly Program Cooperative Research Group. *JAMA* 1996;276:1886-1892.

Cutler JA, Follmann D, Allender PS: Randomized trials of sodium reduction: an overview. *Am J Clin Nutr* 1997;65:643S-651S.

Darné B, Nivarong M, Tugayé A, et al: Hypocaloric diet and antihypertensive drug treatment. A randomized controlled clinical trial. *Blood Press* 1993;2:130-135.

Dyer AR, Elliott P, Shipley M, et al: Body mass index and associations of sodium and potassium with blood pressure in INTERSALT. *Hypertension* 1994;23:729-736.

Eckel RH, Krauss RM: American Heart Association call to action: obesity as a major risk factor of coronary heart disease. *Circulation* 1998;97:2099-2100.

Ehman JW, Ott BB, Short TH: Do patients want physicians to inquire about their spiritual or religious beliefs if they become gravely ill? *Arch Intern Med* 1999;159:1803-1806.

Eliahou H, Iaina A, Gaon T, et al: Body weight reduction to attain normotension in the overweight hypertensive patient. *Int J Obes* 1981;5(suppl 1):157-163.

Estacio RO, Schrier RW: Antihypertensive therapy in type 2 diabetes: Implications of the Appropriate Blood Pressure Control In Diabetes (ABCD) trial. *Am J Cardiol* 1998;82:9R-14R.

Fagan T, Deedwania PC: The cardiovascular dysmetabolic syndrome. *Am J Med* 1998;105:77S-82S.

Ferdinard KC: Substance abuse and hypertension. *J Clin Hypertens* 2000;2:37-40.

Flegal KM, Carroll MD, Kuczmarksi RJ, et al: Overweight and obesity in the United States. Prevalence and trends, 1960-1994. *Int J Obes Relat Met Disord* 1998;22:39-47.

Fletcher EC, DeBehnke RD, Lovoi MS, et al: Undiagnosed sleep apnea in patients with essential hypertension. *Ann Intern Med* 1985;103:190-195.

Garrison RJ, Kannel WB, Strokes J, et al: Incidence and precursors of hypertension in young adults: the Framingham Offspring Study. *Prev Med* 1987;16:235-251.

Goode GK, Miller JP, Heagerty AM: Hyperlipidemia, hypertension, and coronary heart disease. *Lancet* 1995;345:362-364.

Hansson L, Lindholm LH, Niskanen L, et al: Effects of angiotensin-converting-enzyme inhibition compared with conventional therapy on cardiovascular morbidity and mortality in hypertension: the Captopril Prevention Project (CAPP) randomized trial. *Lancet* 1999;353:611-616.

Hansson L, Zanchetti A, Carruthers SG, et al: Effects of intensive blood-pressure lowering and low-dose aspirin in patients with hypertension: principal results of the Hypertension Optimal Treatment (HOT) randomised trial. *Lancet* 1998;351:1755-1762.

Harris MI, Klein R, Cowie CC, et al: Is the risk of diabetic retinopathy greater in non-Hispanic blacks and Mexican Americans than in non-Hispanic whites with type 2 diabetes? A U.S. population study. *Diabetes Care* 1998;21:1230-1235.

Hedblad B, Ogren M, Isacsson SO, et al: Reduced cardiovascular mortality risk in male smokers who are physically active. Results from a 25-year follow-up of the prospective population study of men born in 1914. *Arch Intern Med* 1997;157:893-899.

Himeno E, Nishino K, Nakashima Y, et al: Weight reduction regresses left ventricular mass regardless of blood pressure level in obese subjects. *Am Heart J* 1996;131:313-319.

Hollister LE: Health aspects of cannabis. *Pharmacol Rev* 1986; 38:1-20.

Huber GL, Raines JW: Promoting weight loss in the obese patient. *Patient Care* 2000;34:204-218.

Kales A, Bixler EO, Cadieux RJ, et al: Sleep apnea in a hypertensive population. *Lancet* 1984;2:1005-1008.

Kannel WB, Brand N, Skinner JJ, et al: The relationship of adiposity to blood pressure and development of hypertension. The Framingham Study. *Ann Intern Med* 1967;67:48-59.

Kannel WB, Garrison RJ, Dannenberg AL: Secular blood pressure trends in normotensive persons: the Framingham Study. *Am Heart J* 1993;125:1154-1158.

Kaplan NM: *Clinical Hypertension*, 7th ed. Baltimore, Williams and Wilkins, 1998, p 78.

Kasiske BL, Ma JZ, Kalil RS, et al: Effects of antihypertensive therapy of serum lipids. *Ann Intern Med* 1995;122:133-141.

Klonoff D, Andrews BT, Obana WG: Stroke associated with cocaine use. *Arch Neurol* 1989;46:989-993.

Kotchen TA: Attenuation of hypertension by insulin-sensitizing agents. *Hypertension* 1996;28:219-223.

Kuczmarksi RJ, Carroll MD, Flegal KM, et al: Varying body mass index cutoff points to describe overweight prevalence among U.S. adults: NHANES III (1988 to 1994). *Obes Res* 1997;5:542-548.

Larson DB, Koenig HG: Is God good for your health? The role of spirituality in medical care. *Cleve Clinic J Med* 2000;67:80, 83-84.

Larson DB, Koenig HG, Kaplan BH, et al: The impact of religion on men's blood pressure. *J Relig Health* 1989;28:265-278.

Mänttäri M, Tenkanen L, Manninen V, et al: Antihypertensive therapy in dyslipidemic men. Effects on coronary heart disease incidence and total mortality. *Hypertension* 1995;25:47-52.

McKibbon A, Eady A, Marks S: *PDQ: Evidence-Based Principles and Practices*. Hamilton, Ontario: BC Decker, 1999.

Miller ER Jr, Erlinger TP, Young DR, et al: Lifestyle changes that reduce blood-pressure: implementation in clinical practice. *J Clin Hypertens (Greenwich)* 1999;1:191-198.

Mo W, Singh AK, Arruda JA, et al: Role of nitric oxide in cocaine-induced acute hypertension. *Am J Hypertens* 1998;11:708-714.

Multiple risk factor intervention trial. Risk factor changes and mortality results. Multiple Risk Factor Intervention Trial Research Group. *JAMA* 1982;248:1465-1477.

National Diabetes Information Clearinghouse (NDIC) Diabetes in African Americans. (NIH Publication No. 98-3266 pp 1-7). Bethesda, MD: National Institute of Diabetes and Digestive and Kidney Diseases, National Institutes of Health, 1998.

National High Blood Pressure Education Program Working Group report of primary prevention of hypertension. *Arch Intern Med* 1993;153:186-208.

National High Blood Pressure Education Program Working Group report on hypertension in diabetes. *Hypertension* 1994;23:145-160.

Nazzaro P, Manzari M, Merlo M, et al: Distinct and combined vascular effects of ACE blockade and HMG-CoA reductase inhibition in hypertensive subjects. *Hypertension* 1999;33:719-725.

Nieto FJ, Young TB, Lind BK, et al: Association of sleep disordered breathing, sleep apnea, and hypertension in a large community-based study. Sleep Heart Study. *JAMA* 2000;283:1829-1836.

Osei K, Cottrell DA: Minimal model analyses of insulin sensitivity and glucose-dependent glucose disposal in black and white Americans: a study of persons at risk for type 2 diabetes. *Eur J Clin Invest* 1994;24:843-850.

Poulter NR, Khaw KT, Hopwood BE, et al: The Kenyan Luo migration study: observations on the initiation of a rise in blood pressure. *BMJ* 1990;300:967-972.

Reaven GM: Role of insulin resistance in human disease. *Diabetes* 1988;37:1595-1607.

Reed JW, Shulman NB, Shucker C: *The Black Man's Guide to Good Health*, 1st ed. New York, Berkley Publishing Group, 1994, pp 1-268.

Rexrode KM, Manson JE, Hennekens CH: Obesity and cardiovascular disease. *Curr Opin Cardiol* 1996;11:490-495.

Saunders E, et al: *Cardiovascular Diseases in Blacks,* vol 21. Philadelphia: FA Davis, 1991, pp 56-57.

Sowers JR: Comorbidity of hypertension and diabetes: the Fosinopril Versus Amlodipine Cardiovascular Events Trial (FACET). *Am J Cardiol* 1998;82:15R-19R.

Sowers JR, Reed J: 1999 clinical advisory treatment of hypertension and diabetes. *J Clin Hypertens* 2000;2:132-133.

Staessen J, Fagard R, Lijnen P, et al: Body weight, sodium intake and blood pressure. *J Hypertens* 1989;7(suppl):S19-S23.

Svetkey LP, Simons-Morton D, Vollmer WM, et al: Effects of dietary patterns on blood pressure: subgroup analysis of the Dietary Approaches to Stop Hypertension (DASH) randomized clinical trial. *Arch Intern Med* 1999;159:285-293.

Tatti P, Pahor M, Byington RP, et al: Outcome results of the Fosinopril Versus Amlodipine Cardiovascular Events Randomized Trial (FACET) in patients with hypertension and NIDDM. *Diabetes Care* 1998;21:597-603.

The Seventh Report of the Joint National Committee on Prevention, Detection, Evaluation and Treatment of High Blood Pressure. *JAMA* 2003;289:2560-2572.

Tight blood pressure control and risk of macrovascular and microvascular complications in type 2 diabetes: UKPDS 38. UK Prospective Diabetes Study Group. *Br Med J* 1998;317:703-713.

Tobain L, MacNeill D, Johnson MA, et al: Potassium protection against lesions of the renal tubules, arteries, and glomeruli and nephron loss in salt-loaded hypertensive Dahl S rats. *Hypertension* 1984;6(pt 2):1170-1176.

Wafford MR, Andrew ME, Brown CA, et al: Obesity hypertension in the Atherosclerosis Risk in Communities Cohort: implications of obesity guidelines. *J Clin Hypertens* 1999;1:27-32.

Weinberger MH: *Contemporary Diagnosis and Management of Hypertension*. Newtown, PA, Handbooks in Health Care Co, 1999, p 70.

Weir MR: The role of multiple drug therapy for controlling hypertension in African Americans. *J Clin Hypertens (Greenwich)* 2000; 2:99-108.

Weir MR, Hanes DS: Hypertension in African-Americans: a paradigm of metabolic disarray. *Semin Nephrol* 1996;16:102-109.

Welborn TA, Breckenridge A, Rubinstein AH, et al: Serum-insulin in essential hypertension and in peripheral vascular disease. *Lancet* 1966;1:1336-1337.

Wickelgren I: Obesity: how big a problem? *Science* 1998;280: 1364-1367.

Woods JW, Falk RJ, Pittman AW, et al: Increased red-cell sodium-lithium countertransport in normotensive sons of hypertensive parents. *N Engl J Med* 1982;306:593-595.

Yusuf S, Sleight P, Pogue J, et al: Effects of an angiotensin-converting-enzyme inhibitor, ramipril, on cardiovascular events in high-risk patients. The Heart Outcomes Prevention Study Investigators. *N Engl J Med* 2000;342:145-153.

Zwillich CW: Is untreated sleep apnea a contributing factor for chronic hypertension? *JAMA* 2000;283:1880-1881.

Chapter 4

Target Organ Damage in Hypertensive African Americans

Because African Americans have higher levels of blood pressure, more associated risk factors, and greater delays in diagnosis and treatment, it is not surprising that they have more target organ damage. This increased incidence of target organ damage results in greater morbidity and mortality in African Americans than in whites. African Americans, like whites, have enjoyed a progressive decline in stroke and coronary heart disease mortality since the early 1970s. However, there is no question that excessive hypertension in African Americans is a major contributor to their higher mortality rate, despite the fact that treatment has resulted in some improvement.

Cardiovascular Disease

Left Ventricular Hypertrophy

Savage and his colleagues in the Framingham Heart Study were among the first to show that left ventricular hypertrophy (LVH) is a potent, independent risk factor for cardiovascular morbidity and mortality. Importantly, they found that LVH is statistically independent of age, blood pressure, hypertensive treatment, and other cardiovascular risk factors. Although the electrocardiogram has been the traditional tool for diagnosing LVH (and sug-

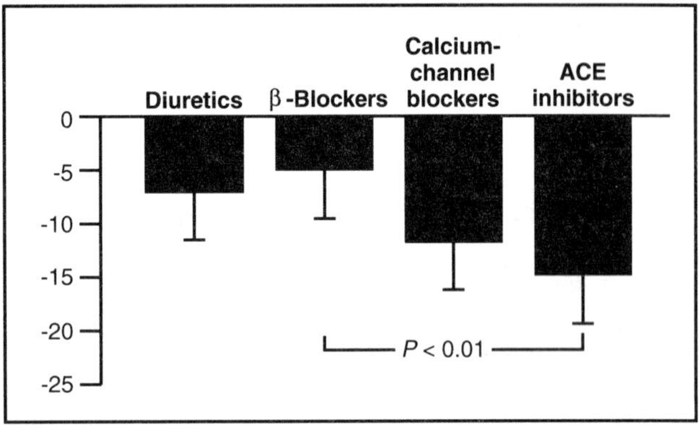

Figure 4-1: Percentage regression of left ventricular hypertrophy by different antihypertension drugs. ACE = angiotensin-converting enzyme. Schmeider et al: *Nephrol Dial Transplant* 1998;13:564-569, by permission of Oxford University Press.

gests that LVH is much more common in blacks than whites), it is not as sensitive in making this diagnosis as the echocardiogram. Most studies suggest that blacks have not only a greater left ventricular wall thickness, but also a greater left ventricular mass, even with equivalent blood pressures. It is becoming increasingly clear that achieving regression of LVH improves cardiovascular risk. Although all drugs that lower blood pressure will regress LVH, it appears that angiotensin-converting enzyme (ACE) inhibitors do it best (Figure 4-1). This is an additional reason to encourage wider use of ACE inhibitors in African Americans. This issue is examined more fully in Chapter 6. However, recent findings show that angiotensin II receptor blockers (ARBs) are effective in reducing morbidity and mortality in hypertensive patients and those with LVH. Results of the Losartan Intervention for Endpoint Reduction in Hypertension (LIFE) study showed significant lowered risk of stroke, myocardial infarction, and new-onset diabetes. Patients in the Valsartan Heart Failure Trial (ValHeFT) were found to have significantly lower morbidity and all-cause mortality.

Coronary Heart Disease

Cardiovascular disease remains the number-one cause of death in the United States. Coronary heart disease accounts for slightly more than one half of deaths from cardiovascular diseases. Although the prevalence of coronary heart disease is suspected to be somewhat less in blacks than in whites, mortality is clearly much higher in black men and women than in their white counterparts. The mortality ratio of blacks compared to whites is even greater in the younger age groups (Table 4-1).

Hypertension, because of its prevalence in blacks and its role as a major risk factor for coronary heart disease, is the number one cause of premature death and disability among African Americans. Confusion continues to exist about the pathogenesis, clinical manifestations, natural history, and therapeutic and diagnostic ramifications of coronary artery disease among African Americans. A study by Peterson et al confirmed what has been suspected for many years: that African Americans are often underdiagnosed and undertreated, both procedurally and surgically, for coronary artery disease. The reasons for the disparity are still being studied.

Heart Failure

Figure 4-2 shows a progressive increase in the percentage of patients with heart failure since 1988. Most patients with heart failure have antecedent or concomitant hypertension. Among African Americans, hypertension is the single most common cause of heart failure. Heart failure is increasing in the general population, but particularly in African Americans because they are prone to concomitant diseases such as diabetes, hypertension, obesity, and ischemic heart disease.

Table 4-1: Death Rates (per 100,000) for Ischemic Heart Disease by Age, Race, and Sex: United States, 1986

	Men	
Age (years)	**White**	**Black**
Ischemic Heart Disease		
	35.8	56.1
35-44	154.3	183.5
45-54	450.1	457.0
55-64	1,062.8	919.4
65-74	2,472.7	1,857.6
0-85+**	169.9	153.9
Acute Myocardial Infarction		
	22.0	31.1
35-44	97.1	101.1
45-54	271.8	247.8
55-64	607.1	492.1
65-74	1,268.0	921.8
0-85+**	94.1	80.5
Chronic Ischemic Heart Disease		
	13.1	23.5
35-44	54.8	77.9
45-54	172.4	200.3
55-64	445.8	409.8
65-74	1,185.4	913.7
0-85+**	74.0	70.6

* Black-white

** Age-adjusted by the direct method, standard: 1940 US population

Women		Ratio*	
White	Black	White	Black
7.1	17.6	1.6	2.5
35.5	80.4	1.2	2.3
147.8	252.3	1.0	1.7
483.9	617.6	0.9	1.3
1,503.0	1,474.9	0.8	1.0
79.5	97.0	0.9	1.2
4.5	9.1	1.4	2.0
22.7	47.3	1.0	2.1
91.4	144.5	0.9	1.6
282.7	335.7	0.8	1.2
747.3	707.4	0.7	0.9
41.7	50.5	0.9	1.2
2.4	8.0	1.8	3.3
12.3	31.7	1.4	2.6
54.6	104.3	1.2	1.9
196.7	272.4	0.9	1.4
745.3	751.6	0.8	1.0
37.1	45.1	1.0	1.2

National Center for Vital Statistics: *Vital Statistics of the United States, 1986. Volume 2. Mortality, Part A.* Washington (DC): US Government Printing Office, 1989. DHHS Publication No. (PHS)89-1101.

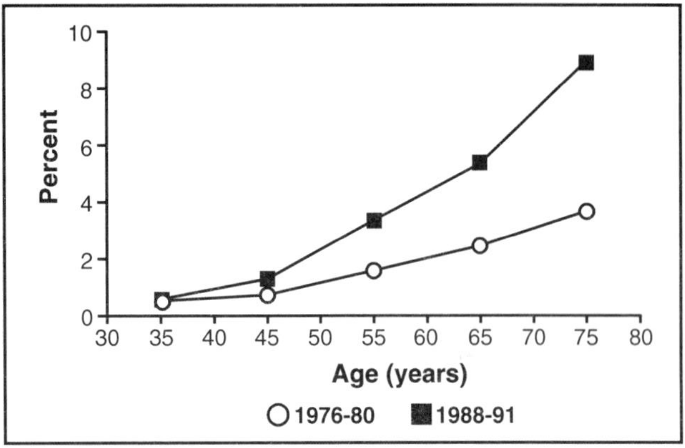

Figure 4-2: Prevalence of heart failure, by age, 1976-1980 and 1988-1991. National Health and Nutrition Examination Survey and National Center for Health Statistics.

Retinopathy

Blood pressure-related changes in the small vessels of the retina can be detected early in hypertension and, therefore, represent a way of assessing vascular disease in other target organs that cannot be seen noninvasively. Because of the increased prevalence of diabetes in African Americans, the concomitant presence of hypertension in this group will likely lead to changes in the optic fundi. Such changes can result in blindness. To a significant degree, aggressive treatment of hypertension and diabetes can prevent this complication.

Peripheral Vascular Disease

Hypertension is a risk factor for aortic aneurysm, dissecting aneurysm, and atherosclerotic disease of peripheral vessels. Although the risk is probably no greater in hypertensive blacks than in hypertensive whites, the concomitant presence of diabetes, dyslipidemia, and cigarette smoking increases it considerably.

Table 4-2: Signs of Stroke

- Sudden weakness or numbness of the face, arm, and leg, especially on one side of the body
- Sudden confusion, trouble speaking or understanding
- Sudden trouble seeing in one or both eyes
- Sudden trouble walking, dizziness, loss of balance or coordination
- Sudden severe headache with no known cause

Cerebrovascular Disease (Stroke)

Clinicians need to know the typical signs of stroke (Table 4-2), especially in hypertensive patients. Hypertension has long been recognized as a risk factor for stroke, with approximately 70% of strokes being attributable to high blood pressure. Treatment of hypertension significantly reduces the risk of stroke, but this reduction is not the same in blacks and whites. Overall, African Americans lag behind whites in the amount of stroke reduction that has been documented.

The effects of treating chronic hypertension differ from the effects of treating high blood pressure detected during an acute stroke.

The treatment of chronic essential hypertension has reduced stroke mortality almost 60% since 1972. The hypertensive patient should always undergo a physical examination, including a neurologic assessment, because some patients will have undiagnosed strokes. The features of stroke in blacks are generally similar to those in whites, but there are some major differences (Table 4-3).

The difference between blacks and whites in the distribution of cerebrovascular disease is especially noteworthy because it indicates that we should consider a different diagnostic workup in each group. For example, black patients may benefit more from transcranial Doppler (TCD) and magnetic resonance angiography (MRA) than from duplex ultrasound, which is used to evaluate extracranial carotid stenosis. Intracranial artery occlusive disease in the larger arteries—which lie outside the brain but still within the skull cavity—and in the branch arteries that penetrate into the brain is more common in African Americans than in whites. The significance of this difference may be that we should approach the diagnosis of cerebrovascular disease somewhat differently in blacks than in whites. Also, this difference could partially explain the higher rate of stroke in blacks.

The treatment of hypertension during an acute stroke is a difficult topic because experts, especially neurologists, often do not agree. Unfortunately, there is little clinical research on this subject. But clinicians can be guided by a few general principles. First, the goal of treatment is to maintain sufficient perfusion to prevent worsening brain ischemia. Second, blood pressure often begins to fall toward prestroke level a few days after the stroke. Third, clinicians should never treat mild-to-moderate hypertension (less than 220/120) unless the blood pressure elevation is accompanied by major organ failure such as acute aortic dissection, myocardial infarction, pulmonary edema, ruptured cerebral aneurysm, or intracranial hemorrhage. Fourth, patients who are candidates for thrombolytic therapy with tissue plasminogen activator (TPA) should maintain a blood pressure lower than 180/110 mm Hg. The goal is to reduce blood pressure by 15% over 24 hours.

No consensus exists about which antihypertensive agents to use, but the ACE inhibitors and the α-blockers (eg, labetalol [Normodyne®, Trandate®]) seem to have favorable hemodynamics regarding autoregulation and intracranial pressure. Nitroprusside (Nitropress®) is easy to titrate, but at least one author has expressed concern about it increasing intracranial pressure.

Table 4-3: Major Differences in Cerebrovascular Disease in African Americans vs Whites

- Hypertension is a vitally important risk factor.
  - Inadequately controlled hypertension accounts for a higher frequency of lacunar infarcts and hypertensive intracerebral hemorrhage in African Americans.
  - Chronic, poorly controlled hypertension contributes to the development of chronic microvascular changes that cause vascular dementia.
- African Americans have a lower frequency of extracranial severe arterial occlusive disease (ie, carotid and vertebral arteries) than similar populations of whites.
- African Americans tend to have a higher frequency of severe intracranial artery occlusive disease than whites.
- Cerebrovascular disease prevalence and mortality rates are higher in African Americans.

Adapted from Gillum RF, Gorelick PB, Cooper ES, eds. *Stroke in Blacks,* 1st ed. Basel, Switzerland: S. Karger AG, 1999.

Many stroke victims are elderly and require special attention because they have impaired systemic baroreceptor responses as well as inadequate cerebral autoregulation. Thus, elderly patients are especially prone to hypotension and even shock during aggressive blood pressure treatment in the presence of an acute stroke, particularly if they have significant extracranial occlusive cerebral vascular disease. Clinicians should carefully consider all of these factors before lowering blood pressure and

Table 4-4: Key Recommendations From the National Stroke Association

1. Treat hypertension to a goal blood pressure of at least < 140/90 mm Hg, but keep in mind that the optimal blood pressure noted in the *Seventh Report of the Joint National Committee on Prevention, Detection, Evaluation, and Treatment of High Blood Pressure* is < 120/80 mm Hg.
2. Post-myocardial infarction patients should receive aspirin and therapy for abnormally high lipid levels.
3. Patients with coronary heart disease and concomitant elevated cholesterol levels or those with any known atherosclerotic disease and concomitant dyslipidemia should receive statins. The National Cholesterol Education Program guidelines for statin therapy should be followed.
4. Patients with carotid artery stenosis of ≥ 60% but < 100% should be considered for endarterectomy by a surgical team with a surgical morbidity and mortality rate of < 3%.

should be aware that different authors often have different recommendations on how to treat these patients.

An acute stroke patient who has normal or even low blood pressure can be particularly challenging, especially if the patient's clinical status is worsening. Some patients will have a significant reversal of their deteriorating neurologic status if their blood pressure is therapeutically elevated. Clinical trials will soon be under way to evaluate this phenomenon. However, to maintain adequate cerebral perfusion in these patients, their blood pressure should be kept at 120 to 150 mm Hg systolic and 60 to 90 mm Hg diastolic or higher, if possible (Table 4-4).

Nephrosclerosis and End-stage Renal Disease

Figure 4-3 shows a staggering increase in the incidence of end-stage renal disease (ESRD) from 1982 to 1995. Although the figures apply to the general population, African Americans appear to be particularly susceptible to renal disease because of hypertension (nephrosclerosis) and other causes. The incidence of nonhypertension-related ESRD among African Americans is more than four times the incidence among whites, according to cases reported to the U.S. Renal Data System. Hypertension-related ESRD in African Americans is much greater for people between 25 and 44 years of age; in fact, the incidence approaches 20 times that of whites. When the increased prevalence of diabetes in African Americans is added to the greater hypertension rate and the combined effect on the kidneys, clinicians can appreciate why this disease is a major public health problem. Because the federal government provides dialysis service to all patients who need it, the total cost of dialysis, combined with lost wages by patients, amounts to a severe economic burden on society.

The treatment of chronic renal insufficiency in hypertensive African Americans is challenging, and the benefits of lowering blood pressure have been controversial until recently because many patients achieving goal blood pressures (ie, < 140/90 mm Hg) have been shown to progress to ESRD despite lower blood pressures.

The Modification of Diet in Renal Disease (MDRD) study examined how dietary modification (low-protein diet) and antihypertensive therapy decreased the progression of renal disease in hypertensive patients. As a result, the African-American Study of Kidney Disease and Hypertension (AASK) was undertaken by the National Institutes of Health. The purpose of the study was to determine the best goal blood pressure (low goal, mean arterial pressure [MAP] < 92 mm Hg, vs usual goal, MAP 102 to 107 mm Hg) to prevent the progression of renal disease.

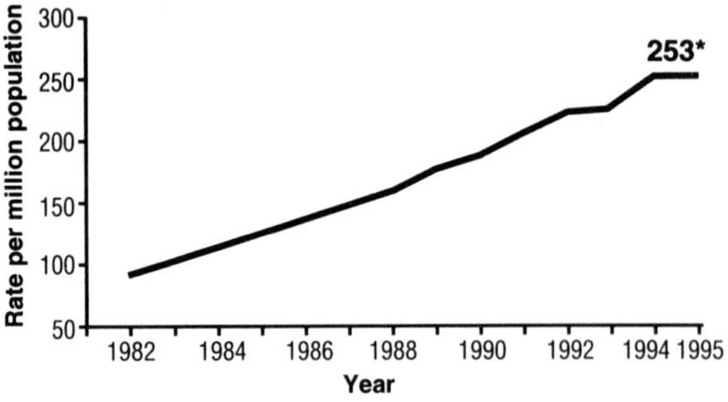

Figure 4-3: Incidence rates per million population of reported end-stage renal disease therapy, 1982-1995, adjusted for age, race, and sex.

In addition, the study was designed to determine the relative renal protectiveness of calcium-channel blockers, β-blockers, and ACE inhibitors. To achieve the desired blood pressure goals, the subject patients required an average of 3.7 drugs (more in the low-goal groups). Diuretics were almost always necessary to achieve goal blood pressures. This is not surprising for a black population, especially one with renal disease. Calcium-channel blockers were used in approximately 62% of patients, regardless of the randomized group. The AASK data and safety monitoring board discontinued the calcium-channel-blocker (amlodipine [Norvasc®]) arm of the study prematurely in hypertensive patients with impaired renal function and proteinuria of 1 g/day or more because the ACE inhibitor arm (ramipril [Altace®]) and the β-blocker arm showed significant reduction in the risks of kidney failure compared to the calcium-channel blocker arm. The study also showed that the standard-target group with a goal blood pressure of 140/90 did not have a further slowing of renal disease pro-

Table 4-5: AASK: Blood Pressure Results

- Patients randomized to standard vs aggressive blood pressure lowering
  - Standard target: 140/90 mm Hg
  - Aggressive target: 125/75 mm Hg
- Aggressive blood pressure lowering beyond usual levels did not further slow renal disease progression
- Findings underscore importance of blood pressure control even in patients with minimal renal dysfunction

AASK = African American Study of Kidney Disease and Hypertension

Adapted from Douglas JG: African American Study of Kidney Disease and Hypertension. American Heart Association Scientific Sessions 2001, November 11-14, 2001, Anaheim, CA.

gression when compared with the aggressive-treatment group with a target blood pressure of 125/75 (Table 4-5).

The results of the AASK study comparisons of metoprolol (Lopressor®, Toprol XL®), a β-blocker, to ramipril and amlodipine were recently released. Figure 4-4 shows the results of these comparisons. As shown, the ACE inhibitor was more effective than the calcium-channel blocker and the β-blocker in reducing the rate of nephropathy progression, but the β-blocker was more effective than the calcium-channel blocker. Further analysis of the study results showed that in addition to slowing the progression of renal disease, the ACE inhibitor reduced other events more effectively compared to the calcium-channel blocker and β-blocker. Thus, in nondiabetic patients with hypertensive nephropathy, ACE inhibitors seem to offer protec-

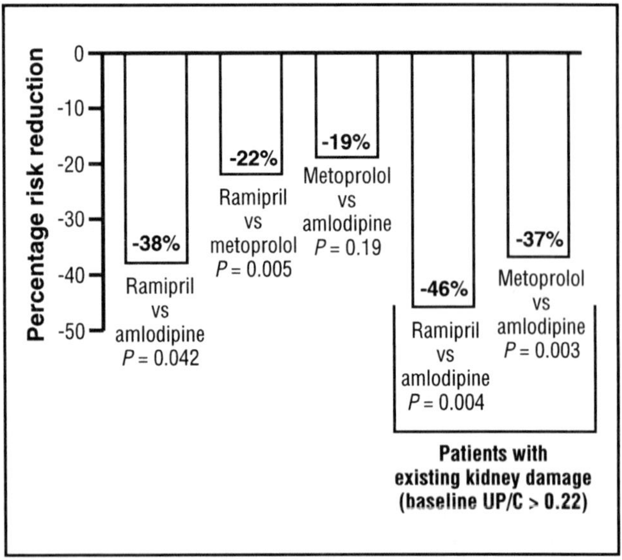

Figure 4-4: African American Study of Kidney Disease and Hypertension: Risk reduction in glomerular filtration rate (GFR) decline, end-stage renal disease, or death with angiotensin-converting enzyme inhibitor, β-blocker, or calcium-channel blocker. Decrease in GFR is from baseline of 50% or 25 mL/min/1.73 m^2. Douglas JG: African American Study of Kidney Disease and Hypertension. American Heart Association Scientific Sessions 2001, November 11-14, 2001, Anaheim, CA.

tion against target organ (kidney) damage independent of their effect on blood pressure. These results are of particular interest because, as stated in Chapter 6, ACE inhibitors were not traditionally thought to be effective in African Americans. In the AASK study, blood pressure was controlled with multiple drugs, but it seems that different combinations of various agents produced different levels of target organ protection. The AASK study may also support earlier initiation of ACE inhibitor and, possibly, angiotensin II receptor blocker

(ARB) therapy to retard or prevent target organ damage in African Americans with severe, complicated hypertension.

At the end of the AASK study, it was concluded that aggressive blood pressure lowering to a target of 125/75 mm Hg did not further slow the progression of renal disease compared to the standard target blood pressure of 140/90 mm Hg. We do not think that this conclusion supports maintaining blood pressure at 140/90 mm Hg if it can be lowered further. It is possible that in AASK, the appropriate use of multiple antihypertensive agents in the group of patients with kidney disease who received an ACE inhibitor produced the maximum achievable benefit in retarding renal disease progression. Thus, further blood pressure lowering could not produce a further benefit.

The implications of this study are consistent with many other studies (eg, Heart Outcomes Prevention Evaluation [HOPE]) of the cardiovascular and renal protectiveness of ACE inhibitors in nondiabetic patients as well as patients with diabetes. This study and others suggest that lowering blood pressure remains paramount for target organ protection and that multiple drug regimens will be required, but that ACE inhibitors appear necessary for maximum target organ protection in high-risk patients.

Recently, ARBs were studied in diabetic, hypertensive patients and were shown to significantly reduce renal dysfunction. These trials are briefly discussed below.

Content Points of Drug Trials in Patients With Diabetes

ACE Inhibitors and Elevated Serum Creatinine in Renal Insufficiency

Often, clinicians are reluctant to use ACE inhibitors in patients with renal insufficiency because elevations in serum creatinine can occur. Bakris and Weir reviewed 12 randomized clinical trials of ACE inhibitors in patients with renal insufficiency at baseline. They found: (1) Any elevations that may occur in patients treated with ACE inhibitors are generally ≤ 30% above baseline, tend to occur within the first 2 weeks of therapy, and stabilize by week 4 of therapy. (2) The most common cause of serum creatinine elevation is a decrease in effective arterial blood volume secondary to aggressive diuresis or to heart failure. (3) Bilateral renal stenosis is a rare cause of serum creatinine elevation and should be suspected if rehydration fails to normalize serum creatinine levels.

Bakris and Weir suggest that ACE inhibitor therapy be stopped only in cases of serum creatinine elevation > 30% above baseline or if serum potassium levels are ≥ 5.6 mmol/L.

Results of PROGRESS

Effect of ACE-inhibitor-based blood pressure lowering in patients with previous stroke/TIA

The Perindopril Protection Against Recurrent Stroke Study (PROGRESS) was a 4-year evaluation of the effects of an ACE-inhibitor-based blood pressure lowering regimen in 6,105 patients with a history of stroke or transient ischemic attack (TIA). Importantly, there were no blood pressure criteria, and patients with a wide range of blood pressures were enrolled. Patients were randomly assigned to active treatment (perindopril [Aceon®] 4 mg ± indapamide [Lozol®] 2.0 to 2.5 mg) or placebo. Active treatment reduced blood pressure by 9/4 mm Hg and reduced stroke risk by 28% ($P < 0.0001$). Significant reductions were also observed in risk of fatal/disabling stroke, nonfatal/nondisabling stroke, ischemic stroke, and cerebral hemorrhage.

Reductions in events by blood pressure status

Subgroup analysis of the PROGRESS results revealed that stroke risk and major vascular risk were reduced similarly in patients classified as nonhypertensive (mean blood pressure at entry 136/79 mm Hg) or hypertensive (> 160/> 90 mm Hg). It was therefore concluded that blood pressure reduction reduces stroke risk in hypertensive and nonhypertensive patients with previous stroke or TIA.

Differing effects of combination and single-drug regimens

Combination therapy (perindopril + indapamide) reduced blood pressure by 12.5 mm Hg and stroke risk by 43% (95% confidence interval [CI] 30% to 54%) vs placebo. Perindopril alone reduced blood pressure by 5/3 mm Hg and stroke risk by 5% (95% CI 19% to 23%) vs placebo. The difference between the two arms was significant ($P < 0.001$, combination vs monotherapy).

Possible explanations for neutral effect of perindopril single-drug therapy

The PROGRESS results for the perindopril-only group are controversial. The PROGRESS investigators argue that the blood pressure reduction achieved (5/3 mm Hg) would be predicted to achieve a reduction in stroke risk of approximately 16% to 20%. While the confidence interval is wide, they believe that the observed risk reduction is "consistent with the moderate effects that would be predicted."

An accompanying editorial by Drs. Jan A. Staessen and Jiguang Wang takes an opposing view. Staessen and Wang state that "blood pressure and random variation do not explain the null results in the perindopril-only group." Based on previous blood pressure lowering trials, they predict a risk reduction of approximately 30% for the blood pressure reduction achieved in the perindopril-only group. Staessen and Wang note that the combination and single-drug groups were not matched, since the responsible physician could specify intensity of treatment. Patients selected for single-drug therapy tended to be lower risk (and, by implication, would have a lower rate of events).

A third possibility, not suggested in the original report or the accompanying editorial, is that the dose of perindopril selected (4 mg) was sufficient to effect a modest reduction in blood pressure but not enough to have clinically significant effects at the vascular wall (the approved dosing interval for perindopril extends to 16 mg).

Recently Completed Studies of ARBs in Patients With Type 2 Diabetes and Renal Disease

The *Seventh Report of the Joint National Committee on Prevention, Detection, Evaluation, and Treatment of High Blood Pressure* (JNC 7) concludes that in patients with type 2 diabetes, hypertension, and microalbuminuria, ACE inhibitors and ARBs have been shown to delay the progression to nephropathy. Furthermore, JNC 7 states that in patients with type 2 diabetes, hypertension, microalbuminuria (> 300 mg/day), nephropathy, or renal insufficiency, an ACE inhibitor or an ARB should be strongly considered. If one class of agents is not tolerated, the other should be substituted. JNC 7 also concludes that the established practice of choosing ACE inhibitors and ARBs as first-line therapy for the prevention of and progression of nephropathy in patients with microalbuminuria or clinical nephropathy is reasonable.

Recently completed clinical trials address the effects of ARBs on the progression of renal disease and cardiovascular outcomes in patients with type 2 diabetes. The Irbesartan Diabetic Nephropathy Trial (IDNT) included 1,715 patients with type 2 diabetes, hypertension, and nephropathy followed up for a mean of 2.6 years. Irbesartan (Avapro®) reduced the primary outcome (composite of ESRD, all-cause mortality, and doubling of baseline serum creatinine concentration) by 20% vs placebo ($P = 0.02$) and by 23% vs amlodipine ($P = 0.006$). Irbesartan reduced progression to ESRD by 23% compared with both treatments ($P = 0.07$ for both comparisons). These effects were not explained by differences in the blood pressures that were achieved. There were no differences between treatment modalities in cardiovascular outcomes or death.

The Reduction of Endpoints in NIDDM with the Angiotensin II Antagonist Losartan (RENAAL) study assessed the effect of losartan (Cozaar®) in 1,513 patients with type 2 diabetes and nephropathy. Patients also received conventional antihypertensive therapy (excluding ACE inhibitors) as needed. Compared with placebo, losartan was associated with a 16% risk reduction in the primary outcome (composite of ESRD, all-cause mortality, and doubling of baseline serum creatinine concentration), $P = 0.02$. It was also associated with a 32% reduction in heart failure hospitalizations.

The Irbesartan Microalbuminuria Type 2 Diabetes in Hypertensive Patients Study (IRMA-2) compared the relative efficacy of irbesartan (150 or 300 mg daily) to that of placebo in 590 patients with type 2 diabetes, hypertension, and microalbuminuria. Compared with placebo, irbesartan was associated with risk reductions in the primary outcome (time to onset of nephropathy) of 39% (150-mg group, $P = 0.08$) and 70% (300-mg group, $P < 0.001$). This study did not assess the impact of treatment on cardiovascular outcomes.

The Microalbuminuria Reduction with Valsartan (MARVAL) study compared the effectiveness of valsartan (Diovan®) and amlodipine in reducing the albumin excretion rate in patients with type 2 diabetes with microalbuminuria. Its conclusions were as follows: (1) In patients with type 2 diabetes and microalbuminuria, arterial blood pressure was reduced to the same extent in the valsartan and amlodipine groups. (2) The albumin excretion rate was significantly reduced in the valsartan group compared with the amlodipine group. (3) Significantly more patients regressed to normoalbuminuria in the valsartan group. (4) The effect of valsartan on the albumin excretion rate was similar in both normotensive and hypertensive subgroups.

Based on several studies, including those mentioned above, the American Diabetes Association (ADA) stated in its 2003 position paper that ACE inhibitors have been shown to delay the progression of nephropathy in patients with type 2 diabetes. In patients with type 2 diabetes with hypertension and microalbuminuria, ACE inhibitors and ARBs have been shown to delay the progression to macroalbuminuria. Also, in patients with type 2 diabetes with

Table 4-6: American Diabetes Association Recommendations for Treatment of Diabetic Nephropathy

Type 1 diabetes with or without hypertension and with any degree of albuminuria:

- ACE inhibitors have been shown to delay the progression of nephropathy

Type 2 diabetes with hypertension and microalbuminuria:

- ACE inhibitors and ARBs have been shown to delay progression to macroalbuminuria

Type 2 diabetes with hypertension, macroalbuminuria, and renal insufficiency:

- ARBs have been shown to delay the progression of nephropathy

If one class of drugs is not tolerated, the other should be substituted.

Adapted from Molitch ME, DeFronzo RA, Franz MJ, et al: Diabetic nephropathy (position statement). *Diabetes Care* 2003;26(suppl 1):S94-S98.

hypertension, macroalbuminuria, and renal insufficiency, ARBs have been shown to delay the progression of nephropathy. When one class of drugs is not tolerated, the other class can be substituted. Serum potassium levels and renal function must be monitored in patients taking either ACE inhibitors or ARBs. These recommendations apply to all patients, including African Americans (Table 4-6).

These studies confirm that ARBs have a renoprotective effect in patients with type 2 diabetes. However, data are lacking on the effects of ARBs on cardiovascular outcomes.

Current Treatment Goals for Diabetes

The most recent treatment goals recommended by the ADA for patients with diabetes are as follows:

- Hemoglobin $A_{1C} < 7\%$
- Blood pressure < 130/80 mm Hg
- Low-density lipoprotein cholesterol < 100 mg/dL
- High-density lipoprotein cholesterol > 45 mg/dL
- Triglycerides < 200 mg/dL

An Approach to Drug Management of Hypertension in Patients With Diabetes

Many patients with diabetes and hypertension will require multidrug therapy to reach their blood pressure goal. ACE inhibitor/diuretic combinations are recommended as initial therapy, based on data showing reduction in cardiovascular events and renal disease progression with each of these classes. If the patient's blood pressure is not at goal, a calcium-channel blocker can be added. If the blood pressure still remains above goal and the patient's pulse rate is ≥ 83 bpm, a β-blocker (or α-β-blocker) can be added. In patients with a lower pulse rate, a second calcium-channel blocker from a different class can be added. If a fifth drug is required, a long-acting α-blocker can be added at bedtime or referral to a hypertension specialist considered.

According to the ADA recommendations, ACE inhibitors are recommended as initial therapy for patients with type 1 diabetes; ACE inhibitors and ARBs are recommended for patients with type 2 diabetes with hypertension and microalbuminuria; and ARBs are recommended for patients with type 2 diabetes with hypertension, macroalbuminuria, and renal insufficiency.

Selected Readings

Agodoa LY, Appel L, Bakris GL, et al: Effect of ramipril vs amlodipine on renal outcomes in hypertensive nephrosclerosis: a randomized controlled trial. *JAMA* 2001;285:2719-2728.

Brenner BM, Cooper ME, de Zeeuw D, et al: Effects of losartan on renal and cardiovascular outcomes in patients with type 2 diabetes and nephropathy. *N Engl J Med* 2001;345:861-869.

Douglas JG: African American Study of Kidney Disease and Hypertension. American Heart Association Scientific Sessions 2001; November 11-14, 2001; Anaheim, CA.

Gillum RF: Cardiovascular disease in the United States: an epidemiologic overview. In: Saunders E, ed. *Cardiovascular Diseases in Blacks*. Philadelphia, FA Davis, 1991, p 3.

Gillum RF, Gorelick PB, Cooper ES, eds. *Stroke in Blacks*, 1st ed. Basel, Switzerland: S. Karger, AG, 1999, pp 1-230.

Gottdeiner JS: Hypertensive heart disease in blacks. In: Saunders E, ed. *Cardiovascular Diseases in Blacks*. Philadelphia, FA Davis, 1991.

Hall WD, Ferrario CM, Moore MA, et al: Hypertension-related mortality in the southeastern United States. *Am J Med Sci* 1997; 313:195-206.

Hall WD, Kusek JW, Kirk KA, et al: Short-term effects of blood pressure control and antihypertensive drug regimen on glomerular filtration rate: the African-American Study of Kidney Disease and Hypertension Pilot Study. *Am J Kidney Dis* 1997;29:720-728.

Hebert LA, Kusek JW, Greene T, et al: Effects of blood pressure control and progressive renal disease in blacks and whites. Modification of Diet in Renal Disease Study Group. *Hypertension* 1997;30:428-435.

Lewis EJ, Hunsicker LG, Clarke WR, et al: Renoprotective effect of the angiotensin-receptor antagonist irbesartan in patients with nephropathy due to type 2 diabetes. *N Engl J Med* 2001;345: 851-860.

Molitch ME, DeFronzo RA, Franz MJ, et al: Diabetic nephropathy (position statement). *Diabetes Care* 2003;26(suppl 1):S94-S98.

Parving HH, Lehnert H, Brochner-Mortensen J, et al: The effect of irbesartan on the development of diabetic nephropathy in patients with type 2 diabetes. *N Engl J Med* 2001;345:870-878.

Peterson ED, Shaw LK, DeLong ER, et al: Racial variation in the use of coronary-revascularization procedures. Are the differences real? Do they matter? *N Engl J Med* 1997;336:480-486.

Savage DD: Echocardiographic left ventricular hypertrophy in blacks. *J Clin Hypertension* 1987;3:615.

Treatment of hypertension in adults with diabetes. *Diabetes Care* 2002;25:199-201.

Chapter **5**

Classification and Evaluation of Hypertensive Patients

Morbidity (target organ dysfunction) and mortality from hypertension are related not only to blood pressure levels, but also to other risk factors and to whether target organ damage is already present. Thus, the *Seventh Report of the Joint National Committee on Prevention, Detection, Evaluation, and Treatment of High Blood Pressure* (JNC 7) includes risk factors in determining treatment strategies for hypertension.

We must emphasize that hypertension is defined by an elevated systolic or diastolic blood pressure above 140/90 mm Hg. This is consistent with data indicating that the systolic blood pressure is as predictive of future cardiovascular events (or more so) as the diastolic blood pressure. Table 6-2 in Chapter 6 combines risk stratification with blood pressure levels as guidelines for the aggressiveness of treatment strategies. This topic is examined in detail in Chapter 6.

Objectives of Evaluation

An important initial step is to confirm that the patient has hypertension. Once this has been done, evaluation is geared toward achieving the following objectives:

- Identification of known secondary causes of high blood pressure

Table 5-1: Proper Measurement of Blood Pressure

Patient Position

- The patient should be seated with the back supported and the arms supported at heart level.
- Blood pressures should be taken in both the supine and upright positions, especially in elderly and diabetic patients.
- Blood pressures should be taken in a quiet room.
- Patients should try to avoid confounding factors such as tobacco, alcohol, and caffeine.

Equipment

- A mercury sphygmomanometer, a calibrated aneroid manometer, or a validated electronic device. The bladder within the cuff should encircle at least 80% of the arm; a cuff that is too large will give falsely low readings, and a cuff that is too small will give falsely high readings.
- Stethoscope—use the bell of the stethoscope.

- Assessment for the presence or absence of target organ damage and cardiovascular disease, including determining the extent of disease and the response to therapy
- Identification of other cardiovascular risk factors or concomitant disorders that may define prognosis and guide treatment

Patient assessment should also include a history of recent changes in weight, physical activity, or tobacco use; dietary assessment for intake of alcohol, sodium, fat, and caffeine; history of any over-the-counter medications or herbal remedies; history of illicit drug use; efficacy and side effects of previous antihypertensive therapy; and in-

Technique

- Inflate the bladder quickly to a blood pressure of 20 mm Hg above the systolic pressure, which is determined by the disappearance of the palpated radial pulse during bladder inflation.
- Allow bladder to deflate at 2 mm Hg/sec.
- Record Korotkoff phase I (appearance of sound) and phase V (disappearance of sound) as the systolic and diastolic, respectively.

Other Issues

- If blood pressure is elevated (ie, > 140/90 mm Hg), do blood pressure measurements in the legs.
- If blood pressure is consistently higher in one arm, use that reading and consider potential reasons for the difference (eg, aneurysms, artifact).

formation on psychosocial and socioeconomic issues (ie, family structure, place of residence, employment status, and educational level).

Steps in Evaluation of Hypertensive Patients

Although the actual diagnosis of hypertension is largely an objective measurement, other pertinent medical data should be obtained from all patients.

Complete Medical History

A medical history should include any information on blood pressures obtained in the past and a history of symptoms of heart disease, cerebrovascular disease, renal disease, peripheral vascular disease, dyslipidemia, diabetes, gout, sexual dysfunction, or other comorbid conditions. One simple question to ask is: "Do you think you know why your blood pressure is up?" This question will not only reveal important clinical information, but also give you insight into how educated the patient is about hypertension.

Physical Examination and Laboratory and Ancillary Studies

Any evaluation of a patient with documented hypertension should have three goals: (1) to identify known causes of hypertension (ie, secondary hypertension); (2) to determine the presence or absence of target organ damage, the extent of disease, and the response to therapy; and (3) to identify cardiovascular risk factors or comorbid conditions that could influence hypertension prognosis, diagnosis, or treatment. The first part of any physical includes the vital signs, with the blood pressure measurement obtained by proper methods (Table 5-1). The remaining elements of the physical examination are listed in Table 5-2.

Unfortunately, laboratory and ancillary studies are under constant surveillance by third-party payers, making it difficult for clinicians to order tests they believe are necessary. Therefore, clinicians should be aware of the routine tests recommended by the *Sixth Report of the Joint National Committee on Prevention, Detection, Evaluation, and Treatment of High Blood Pressure,* which include complete blood count, urinalysis, blood chemistry (potassium, sodium, fasting glucose, creatinine, total cholesterol, and high-density lipoprotein [HDL] cholesterol), thyroid stimulating hormone, and, in carefully selected patients, echocardiography to assess left ventricle size.

Other tests may be helpful in specific clinical situations, such as plasma renin, urinary catecholamines, and

Table 5-2: Physical Examination of the Hypertensive Patient

- Measure blood pressure, preferably with mercury sphygmomanometer.
- Determine height, weight, and waist circumference.
- Use funduscopy to evaluate for hypertensive retinopathy.
- Auscultate the neck for carotid or thyroid bruits; palpate for thyroid size and for distended veins.
- Assess heart rate, rhythm, size; auscultate for murmurs, 3rd and 4th heart sounds.
- Listen to the lungs for rales, wheezes, rhonchi, distant breath sounds.
- Evaluate abdomen for bruits, organomegaly, and abnormal aortic pulsation.
- Evaluate extremities for edema and for diminished or absent pulses.
- Perform a neurologic examination.

the captopril renal scan in suspected secondary hypertension. In a patient with suspected vascular disease, examination of structural alterations by ultrasound, by intravenous arteriography, or by flow characteristic by magnetic resonance angiography (MRA) may confirm or exclude the presence of disease, potentially changing the management of blood pressure. However, up to 95% of hypertensive African Americans will have primary (ie, essential) hypertension; therefore, in many patients, looking for secondary causes will be time-consuming and costly if there is no justifiable reason to suspect secondary hypertension.

Table 5-3: Factors Affecting the Immediate Accuracy of Office BP

Increases Recorded BP

Examinee

Pseudohypertension
White-coat reaction
  To physician
  To nonphysician
Paretic arm (due to stroke)
Pain, anxiety
Acute smoking
Acute caffeine ingestion
Acute ethanol ingestion
Distended bladder
Talking; singing

Setting, equipment

Environment noise
Leaky bulb valve
Blocked manometer vents
Cold hands on stethoscope

Examiner

Expectation bias
Impaired hearing

Examination

Cuff too narrow
Cuff not centered
Cuff over clothing
Elbow too low
Cuff too low
Too short rest period
Back unsupported
Arm unsupported
Too slow deflation
Parallax error
Using phase IV (adult)
Cold season (vs warm)

Decreases BP

Examinee

Recent meal
Missed auscultatory gap
High stroke volume
Habituation
Shock

Setting, equipment

Noisy environment
Faulty aneroid device
Low mercury level
Leaky bulb

Examiner

Reading to next lowest 5 or 10 mm Hg, or expectation bias
Impaired hearing

Examination

Noisy environment
Left vs right arm
Resting for too long (25 min)
Elbow too high
Deflation too rapid
Excess bell pressure
Parallax error (aneroid)

No Effect on BP

Examinee

Menstrual phase
Chronic caffeine ingestion
Phenylephrine nasal spray
Cuff self-inflation

Examinee and Examiner

Discordance in sex or race

Examination

Thin shirtsleeve under cuff
Bell vs diaphragm
Cuff inflation per se
Hour or day
(during work hours)
Room temperature

BP = blood pressure

Modified from Kaplan NM: *Clinical Hypertension,* 7th ed. Baltimore, Williams and Wilkins, 1998, p 21.

Confirmation of Diagnosis for Hypertensive Patients

When you stop and think about how often we make clinical decisions based on a patient's blood pressure, it is amazing how little time we spend teaching the proper technique for recording an accurate blood pressure level. First, the patient must be told that the diagnosis of hypertension is a process, not a single measurement. The patient should have three readings at least 1 week apart, and least two readings should be taken on each visit. If the reading is consistently higher in one arm than in the other, the higher blood pressure reading should be used to determine the diagnosis and treatment. According to JNC 7, hypertension can be diagnosed if the systolic blood pressure is 140 mm Hg or greater, the diastolic blood pressure is 90 mm Hg or greater, or the patient is already taking antihypertensive medication. Guidelines for the proper measurement of blood pressure are listed in Table 5-1. Factors affecting the accuracy of blood pressure measurement are listed in Table 5-3.

If the diagnosis is still difficult to determine because the patient has white-coat hypertension or extremely labile blood pressure, 24-hour ambulatory blood pressure monitoring can be helpful. The ambulatory monitor is often more helpful than home self-monitoring because it is less subject to operator bias and gives nocturnal blood pressure readings. A hypertension specialist certified by the American Society of Hypertension can assist with monitor interpretation. Also, by evaluating the patient for target organ damage, the clinician can obtain good circumstantial evidence that the patient has sustained hypertension vs episodic hypertension. The main point to remember about diagnosing hypertension is that it is no longer acceptable to give a diagnosis of borderline hypertension. According to JNC 7, all patients should be given a definitive diagnosis of normotension, prehypertension, or hypertension.

Selected Readings

Kaplan NM: *Clinical Hypertension,* 7th ed. Lippincott Williams and Wilkins, 1998, p 122.

Mänttäri M, Tenkanen L, Manninen V, et al: Antihypertensive therapy in dyslipidemic men. Effects on coronary heart disease incidence and total mortality. *Hypertension* 1995;25:47-52.

Seventh Report of the Joint National Committee on Prevention, Detection, Evaluation, and Treatment of High Blood Pressure (JNC-VII). *JAMA* 2003;289:2560-2572.

Chapter 6

Treatment of Hypertension in African Americans

Lifestyle Modifications

The *Seventh Report of the Joint National Committee on Prevention, Detection, Evaluation, and Treatment of High Blood Pressure* (JNC 7) uses the word *prevention* in its title, thereby emphasizing the potential of lifestyle modifications to prevent hypertension.

The lifestyle modifications listed in Table 6-1 have proven to be effective in reducing blood pressure and other cardiovascular risk factors at little cost or risk. Clinicians should encourage all their hypertensive patients to adopt these lifestyle changes. However, because of the unique features of hypertensive African Americans, the International Society on Hypertension in Blacks has recently recommended and published a modified protocol for the pharmacologic and nonpharmacologic treatment of hypertension in African Americans. As our population becomes more overweight, many health care providers contend that lifestyle education should start in adolescence, ideally before obesity occurs because of poor lifestyle choices. It is also important to tell patients already on antihypertensive therapy that following these lifestyle modifications can help minimize the number and dosage of antihypertensive medications needed to reach their goal blood pressure. The Dietary Approaches to Stop Hypertension (DASH) diet has been examined in Chapter 3, and while physicians acknowledge that a significant number of patients will not follow dietary instructions, even a partial change in habits can help to lower blood pressure. The behavioral changes needed to successfully adopt lifestyle changes are not easily achieved and require an ongoing team approach, which will be discussed in Chapter 7.

Pharmacologic Treatment

Failure to respond to lifestyle modifications for hypertension within a reasonable time frame will lead to the need for pharmacologic management. Factors to consider before prescribing antihypertension drugs include the degree of blood pressure elevation, the presence of target organ damage or dysfunction, and the presence of other risk factors that may potentiate the effect of elevated blood pressure. The more factors that exist, the higher the risks are for hypertension, so treatment will probably be more aggressive. African Americans are likely to have multiple risk factors, in addition to socioeconomic issues, that can affect overall outcome.

Numerous studies have shown that reducing blood pressure with drugs decreases cardiovascular morbidity and mortality. This has been shown for stroke, coronary events, and renal disease, in addition to hypertension and all-cause mortality. These benefits have been shown in African Americans regardless of blood pressure level, age, or socioeconomic status.

Although the overall goal is to reduce cardiovascular morbidity and mortality by lowering blood pressure to less than 140/90 mm Hg, high-risk populations, such as patients in risk category C, require even lower goals (Table 6-2). Although the data are not in, we and several of our colleagues believe that African-American hypertensives represent a high-risk population—analogous to diabetic patients, older persons, and other patients with multiple risk factors—that should be treated to achieve lower goals, specifically < 130/80 mm Hg. Chapter 2 describes the patho-

Table 6-1: Lifestyle Modifications to Manage Hypertension*

Modification	Recommendation
Weight reduction	Maintain normal body weight (BMI, 18.5-24.9)
Adopt DASH eating plan	Consume a diet rich in fruits, vegetables, and low-fat dairy products, with a reduced content of saturated and total fat
Dietary sodium reduction	Reduce dietary sodium intake to no more than 100 mEq/L (2.4 g sodium or 6 g sodium chloride)
Physical activity	Engage in regular aerobic physical activity such as brisk walking (at least 30 minutes per day, most days of the week)
Moderation of alcohol consumption	Limit consumption to no more than 2 drinks/day (1 oz or 30 mL ethanol [eg, 24 oz beer, 10 oz wine, or 3 oz 80-proof whiskey]) in most men and no more than 1 drink/day in women and lighter-weight persons.

BMI = body mass index calculated as weight in kg divided by the square of height in meters; BP = blood pressure; DASH = Dietary Approaches to Stop Hypertension

*For overall cardiovascular risk reduction, stop smoking. The effects of implementing these modifications are dose- and time-dependent and could be higher for some individuals.

Approximate Systolic BP Reduction, Range
5-20 mm Hg/10-kg weight loss
8-14 mm Hg
2-8 mm Hg
4-9 mm Hg

National Heart, Lung, and Blood Institute: *JNC 7 Express: The Seventh Report of the Joint National Committee on Prevention, Detection, Evaluation, and Treatment of High Blood Pressure.* Rockville, MD, US Department of Health and Human Services; May 2003. NIH Publication no. 03-5233.

Table 6-2: Classification and Management of Blood Pressure in Adults ≥ 18 Years

Blood Pressure Classification
Normal (<120/80 mm Hg)
Prehypertension (120-139/80-89 mm Hg)
Stage 1 hypertension (140-159/90-99 mm Hg)
Stage 2 (≥ 160 [systolic] or ≥ 100 [diastolic] mm Hg

ACE = angiotensin-converting enzyme;
ARB = angiotensin-receptor blocker

*Compelling indications include diabetes, chronic kidney disease, heart failure, postmyocardial infarction, high risk of coronary disease, and stroke.

physiologic profile of the hypertensive African-American patient. Several of the factors in this profile suggest that endothelial dysfunction (a precursor of atherosclerosis) may occur at an earlier stage in hypertensive African Americans. Thus, the therapeutic implications suggest a revision

Management and Initial Drug Therapy

Encourage lifestyle modification.

No drug indicated except for patients with chronic kidney disease or diabetes to reach a BP goal of < 130/80 mm Hg.

Encourage lifestyle modification.

Diuretics for most; may consider ACE inhibitor, ARB, β-blocker, or calcium-channel blocker, or combination.

Drugs for those with compelling indications*; other antihypertensive drugs as needed

Encourage lifestyle modification for all.

Combination of two drugs for most patients (thiazide-type diuretic and ACE inhibitor or ARB or β-blocker or calcium-channel blocker**)

Drugs for those with compelling indications; other antihypertensive drugs as needed.

Encourage lifestyle modification for all.

**Initial combined drug therapy should be used cautiously in those at risk for orthostatic hypotension.

Modified from The Seventh Report of the Joint Committee on Prevention, Detection, Evaluation, and Treatment of High Blood Pressure. *JAMA* 2003;289:2560-2572.

of the usual strategies. The International Society on Hypertension in Blacks has recently published such a revision, which is addressed below and summarized in Figure 6-1. A study in progress, Consequences of the Reversal of Endothelial Dysfunction With Use of Quinapril (CONQUER), is testing hypertensive African Americans at baseline for endothelial dysfunction (flow-mediated vasodilatation) and retesting after treatment with a tissue-avid angiotensin-converting enzyme (ACE) inhibitor (quinapril [Accupril®]). The hypothesis is that ACE inhibition may improve endothelial dysfunction in high-risk patients, independent of its blood pressure-lowering effect. The Heart Outcomes Prevention Evaluation (HOPE) Study (discussed in Chapter 3) has clearly shown that high-risk patients do better with ACE-inhibitor therapy (ramipril [Altace®]) compared to placebo. This will be discussed further when we examine specific drugs later in this chapter.

The algorithm proposed by JNC 7 for the treatment of hypertension indicates that after a trial of lifestyle modification, the initial drugs of choice for uncomplicated hypertension should be thiazide-type diuretics for most patients or consideration of ACE inhibitor, ARB, β-blocker, or calcium-channel blocker or combination (stage 1) or 2-drug combination of diuretic and ACE inhibitor or ARB or β-blocker or calcium-channel blocker (stage 2). These recommendations are based on the fact that these drugs have been shown in long-term, randomized, controlled trials to reduce cardiovascular morbidity and mortality. However, other drugs are recommended when compelling indications exist to use them, such as when data show benefit over diuretics and other antihypertensive agents. Figure 6-2 summarizes these recommendations.

In African Americans, diuretics have proven to be quite effective (as they have in whites) in lowering blood pressure. This is consistent with the volume-dependent, salt-sensitive, and low-renin form of hypertension often found in blacks. Doses greater than the equivalent of 25 mg of hydrochlorothiazide (Esidrix®, HydroDIURIL®, Microzide®, Oretic®) may be associated with more clinical side effects and metabolic electrolyte disturbances and may not lower blood pressure as much as doses of 25 mg or less.

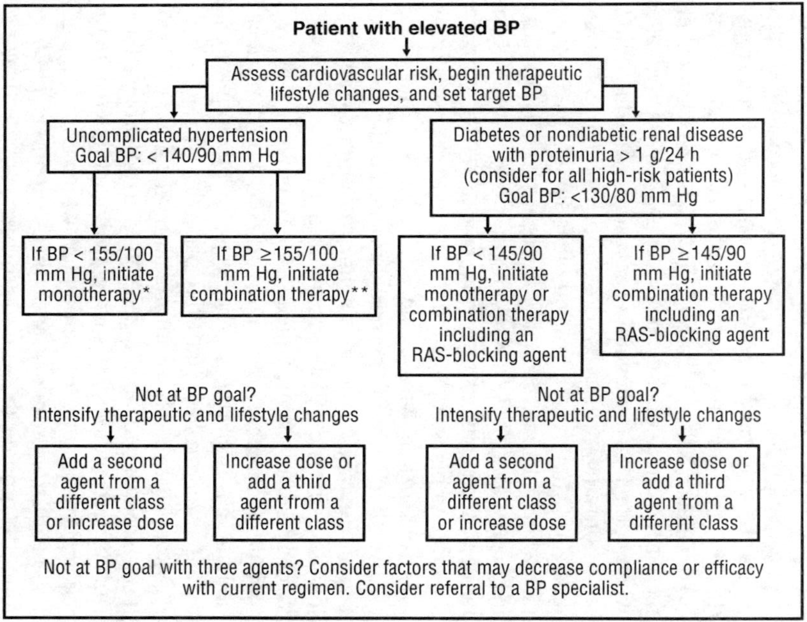

Figure 6-1: Critical algorithm for achieving goal blood pressure (BP) in hypertensive African Americans. * Initiate monotherapy at the recommended starting dose with an agent from any of the following classes: diuretics, β-blockers, calcium-channel blockers (CCBs), angiotensin-converting enzyme (ACE) inhibitors, or angiotensin II receptor blockers (ARBs). ** Initiate low-dose combination therapy with any of the following combinations: β-blocker/diuretic, ACE inhibitor/CCB, ARB/diuretic. RAS = renin-angiotensin system. Douglas JG, et al, *Arch Intern Med* 2003;163:525-541.

There has been considerable discussion about the relative efficacy of other antihypertensive drugs in African Americans compared to whites. African Americans have long been known to have a higher prevalence of hypertension than whites, and this hypertension has been found to be especially responsive to certain classes of antihypertensives. The calcium antagonists have good efficacy in blacks, with a recent South African study showing that a dihydropyridine calcium antagonist (the nifedipine [Adalat®, Procardia®] gastrointestinal therapeutic system) was more effective than a thiazide diuretic, an ACE inhibitor, and even a nondihydropyridine calcium antagonist. In the United States, the Veterans Affairs Cooperative Study Group found that the calcium antagonist diltiazem (Cardizem®, Cartia XT®, Dilacor XR®, Diltia XT®, Tiazac®) was the most effective hypertension drug in African Americans of all ages when compared to atenolol (Tenormin®), thiazide diuretics, clonidine (Catapres®), captopril (Capoten®), and prazosin (Minipress®). Several other studies have shown that while calcium-channel blockers are equally effective in hypertensive blacks and whites, the β-blockers, ACE inhibitors, and angiotensin-receptor blockers (ARBs) are less effective in blacks compared to whites at the usual doses prescribed. As shown in Table 6-3, increased dosing (especially with ACE inhibitors) results in significantly improved response in blacks. Dietary sodium restriction and adding a low-dose diuretic will also result in an improved response, similar to that in white patients. Also, combining an ACE inhibitor with a calcium-channel blocker, with or without a diuretic, has been found to be very effective in managing hypertension in black and white patients.

In view of the above information on calcium antagonists, research into the new generation of dihydropyridines, such as lercanidipine, has generated much interest in the medical community. Lercanidipine, which is awaiting US Food and Drug Administration (FDA) approval, has been found to provide the same antihypertensive efficacy as amlodipine (Norvasc®) and felodipine (Plendil®) with a lower incidence of peripheral edema. The lower incidence of peripheral edema is particularly important because edema tends to be dose dependent and is a major reason for discontinuation of the dihydropyridines as a class. In the COHORT study, researchers compared the new dihydropyridines lercanidipine 10 mg daily and lacidipine 2 mg daily with amlodipine 5 mg daily. After 6 months, all groups showed similar reductions in blood pressure. The lercanidipine and lacidipine groups showed no statistically significant difference in the incidence of edema. The amlodipine group had a 18.5% incidence of edema, compared to a 7.5% incidence in the lercanidipine group. Perhaps more importantly, the early discontinuation because of edema was 8.3% in the amlodipine group vs 1.9% in the lercanidipine group. Ongoing research may prove that lercanidipine has a different impact on the sympathetic nervous system compared to amlodipine. We can expect that more research will be done with this new subset of calcium antagonists in cohorts of mostly African-American patients.

Two community-based hypertension studies involved significant numbers of African Americans and may have an important impact on how this population is treated in the future. The Antihypertensive and Lipid Lowering Treatment to Prevent Heart Attack Trial (ALLHAT) was designed to help determine whether the newer agents (calcium-channel blockers, ACE inhibitors, and α-blockers) had a long-term benefit on cardiovascular disease comparable to that of diuretics. The α-blocker arm of the trial was discontinued because of the failure of the selected α-blocker (doxazosin [Cardura®]) to reduce cardiovascular events as well as the diuretic chlorthalidone (Hygroton®, Thalitone®).

The other trial is the African-American Study of Kidney Disease and Hypertension (AASK). This study was designed to determine if much lower goal blood pressures are better than higher-goal blood pressures (mean 92 to

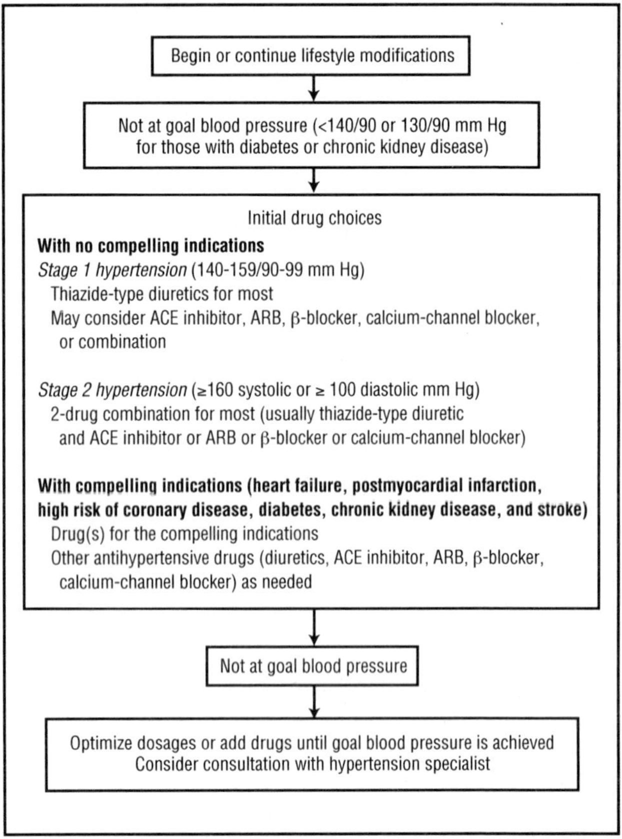

Figure 6-2: Algorithm for the treatment of hypertension. Modified from The Seventh Report of the Joint Committee on Prevention, Detection, Evaluation, and Treatment of High Blood Pressure. *JAMA* 2003;289:2560-2572.

102 mm Hg) and if combinations of specific antihypertensive drugs are better in preventing end-stage renal disease in high-risk, renally impaired hypertensive African Americans. Subjects in this study were given three to five

Table 6-3: Comparative Efficacy of a β-Blocker, a Calcium-Channel Blocker, and an ACE Inhibitor in Hypertensive Blacks

	Atenolol	Captopril	Verapamil SR
Period 2 (N=345*)			
N	118	112	115
Success %	55.1	43.8	65.2
Failure %	44.9	56.3	34.8
Period 3 (low and high dose) (N=307*)			
N	109	98	100
Success %	59.6	57.1	73.0
Failure %	40.4	42.9	27.0
Period 3 (high dose only) (N=157*)			
N	56	47	54
Success %	58.9	61.7	83.3
Failure %	41.1	38.3	16.7

*Numbers of patients given are numbers for whom data are available.

Saunders et al: *Arch Intern Med* 1990;150:1707-1713. Reprinted with permission.

drugs in combination. This study and its recently released results are described in Chapter 4.

The ALLHAT trial was largely driven by a high percentage of African Americans (35%). Its major conclusions were that (1) goal blood pressures are achievable in most hypertensive patients, (2) thiazide-type diuretics are the preferred first step in treatment of hypertension in most patients, and (3) combination therapy that includes a diuretic will be required in most patients with hypertension. The AASK trial confirmed that the ACE inhibitor ramipril is significantly more effective than the dihydropyridine amlodipine and slightly more effective than the β-blocker atenolol in slowing the progression of hypertensive renal disease. AASK also found that the lower goal blood pressure of 125/75 mm Hg was no more effective than 140/90 mm Hg in this regard.

Studies on risk factors that cause endothelial dysfunction resulting in processes leading to atherosclerosis may be of special interest to hypertensive African Americans. The ongoing CONQUER trial is such an example. In this study, the investigators hypothesize that endothelial dysfunction is present earlier in African Americans with stage 1 or 2 hypertension (compared to whites) and may precede the development of clinically apparent vascular disease or target organ damage. An up-regulated tissue, the renin-angiotensin-aldosterone system (RAAS), may be responsible. Thus, treatment with ACE inhibitors (independent of blood pressure lowering) may improve flow mediator vasodilation (ie, endothelial dysfunction). The study is ongoing. Investigators have speculated that lowering blood pressure is a necessary, but not sufficient, step to reduce the global risk of high-risk (ie, African-American) hypertensive patients. Thus, it appears that treating the partial indicator (elevated blood pressure) is necessary to reduce cardiovascular morbidity and mortality, but more could be achieved by also treating the underlying problem (endotheliopathy). JNC 7 confirmed this clinical principle for diabetic patients with nephropathy, in whom ACE inhibitors or ARBs were recommended as 'compelling' therapy. Likewise, ACE inhibitors or other antihypertensive agents are recommended for certain cardiovascular problems, and β-blockers, ACE inhibitors, and aldosterone antagonists are recommended for post-myocardial infarction patients (with left ventricular dysfunction) and those with ischemic syndromes. Consequently, a new paradigm is indicated for the management of high-risk hypertensive patients, such as African Americans, in whom factors beyond blood pressure control (eg, endothelial dysfunction, vascular compliance) must be addressed with the appropriate therapy to achieve the best outcomes. Figure 6-3 is a compilation algorithm the authors suggest for the treatment of hypertension in African Americans. In its Consensus Statement on the Management of High Blood Pressure in African Americans, published in the March 10, 2003, issue of the *Archives of Internal Medicine*, the International Society on Hypertension in Blacks recommended a similar protocol. It also suggested a lower goal blood pressure (< 130/80 mm Hg) for African Americans and initiation of combination therapy for patients at higher risk as indicated by blood pressure level (≥ 155/100 mm Hg) or by comorbidities such as diabetes or renal disease. An algorithm including these recommendations is presented in Figure 6-1.

Thus far, the ACE inhibitor and the ARB trials seem to address the issue of treating risk factors beyond high blood pressure and should therefore be used more frequently in hypertensive African Americans, independent of their blood pressure-lowering effects. The HOPE study (although it had very few African Americans) and the early results from the AASK study (see Chapter 4) certainly are consistent with this recommendation. However, we must again emphasize that blood pressure control is paramount in the effort to reduce cardiovascular morbidity and mortality. Other drugs (diuretics, calcium-channel blockers, vasodilators, adrenergic blockers, etc) are often needed in combination with an ACE inhibitor or an ARB to achieve goal blood pressure.

ACE-inhibitor-induced cough has been found to be more common in African Americans than in whites. In contrast, ARBs have consistently been found to have a side effect profile no greater than that of placebo. Therefore, an ARB may become an important addition to the antihypertensive regimen of African Americans in the near future.

A New Paradigm for Treating Patients With Type 2 Diabetes

Results of recent clinical trials such as the Irbesartan in Diabetic Nephropathy Trial (IDNT), the Irbesartan in Patients With Type 2 Diabetes and Microalbuminuria (IRMA-2) study, and the Reduction of Endpoints in NIDDM With the Angiotensin II Antagonist Losartan (RENAAL) trial support physicians' already common practice of using ARBs in patients with type 2 diabetes with nephropathy. The IDNT trial findings revealed that the ARB irbesartan (Avapro®) was superior to amlodipine in reducing the primary composite end point (doubling of serum creatinine, development of end-stage renal failure, and all-cause mortality). This was significant because the amlodipine and conventional treatment groups were designed so that the blood pressure lowering effects in the different groups would be similar; however, this did not result in a same degree of renal protection for each group. The IRMA-2 trial involved patients with type 2 diabetes with microalbuminuria and found that irbesartan significantly reduced the proportion of patients that developed overt nephropathy: 14.9% of the placebo group developed overt renal disease vs 5.2% of the irbesartan 300 mg group. The investigators were particularly interested in the dose-dependent nature of the renal protection, as shown by the progression to overt nephropathy in 9.7% of the 150-mg irbesartan group vs only 5.2% of the 300-mg dose cohort. The RENAAL trial, a diabetic nephropathy study that investigated the effect of losartan (Cozaar®) on the primary composite end point (doubling of serum creatinine, end-stage renal disease, and death), found that ARB therapy (losartan) was superior to conventional therapy, which consisted of β-blockers, diuretics, or calcium-channel blockers, but not ACE inhibitors. The Losartan Intervention for Endpoint Reduction in Hypertension (LIFE) study studied 9,193 patients with hypertension and evidence of left ventricular hypertrophy by electrocardiography. Its findings included a reduction in overall cardiovascular morbidity and mortality (mainly stroke vs myocardial infarction) and a 25% reduction in new onset diabetes in the losartan group vs the atenolol group. This second, unexpected finding gives even more support to the practice of using ARBs in patients with hypertension who are at high risk for developing diabetes.

Should diabetic African-American patients with hypertension be treated any differently? Clinicians should be aware that African Americans appear to be particularly susceptible to end-stage renal disease, as noted in Chapter 4 of this book, which strongly suggests that clinicians should move quickly and aggressively when treating this high-risk population. Also, ARBs, like ACE inhibitors, generally need to be dosed higher in African Americans in order to achieve the same antihypertensive efficacy found in similar white populations. Prior data with the ARB tasosartan (which is now unavailable due to safety concerns) suggested that African-American patients required doses three times higher than those of their white counterparts in order to achieve comparable blood pressure responses. African Americans were also found to respond differently to ARBs in the LIFE trial, with losartan being found to be less effective than atenolol. Of the 533 black patients in the LIFE trial, those in the atenolol-based cohort had a lower risk of cardiovascular death, myocardial infarction, and stroke than those in the losartan group, despite similar blood pressure lowering with both drugs. As with many other antihypertensive medications, the blood pressure reduction achievable with ARBs can be significantly increased by adding a diuretic. Researchers are also beginning to study the effects of combining ACE inhibitors and ARBs.

Begin or continue lifestyle modifications

- Weight reduction
- Regular aerobic physical activity
- Reduction of dietary sodium
- Adequate dietary potassium, calcium, magnesium
- Reduction of dietary saturated fats and cholesterol
- Moderation of alcohol intake
- Discontinuation of tobacco use
- Reduction of stress

Not at goal blood pressure (<130/85)

Initial Drug Choices (specific indications and utility in African Americans)*

- ACE inhibitors—heart failure, diabetes with microalbuminuria, renal disease with heavy proteinuria, MI with systolic dysfunction and high-risk hypertensives
- Angiotensin-receptor blockers (ARBs)—recommended when ACE inhibitors are not tolerated, but can be used in monotherapy
- α-blockers—recommended in combination with other antihypertensive agents or for concomitant prostatism
- α-β-blockers—more effective than β-blockers in monotherapy but more effective in combination with diuretics
- Calcium antagonists—very effective in monotherapy or in combination with other agents
- Diuretics—very effective in monotherapy or in combination with most other agents; low doses recommended to decrease adverse drug effects

* For all of the above, start with low dose of long-acting, once-daily drug and titrate to maximum tolerated or recommended dose. In some cases, initial drug therapy may be a combination of synergistic and additive drugs.

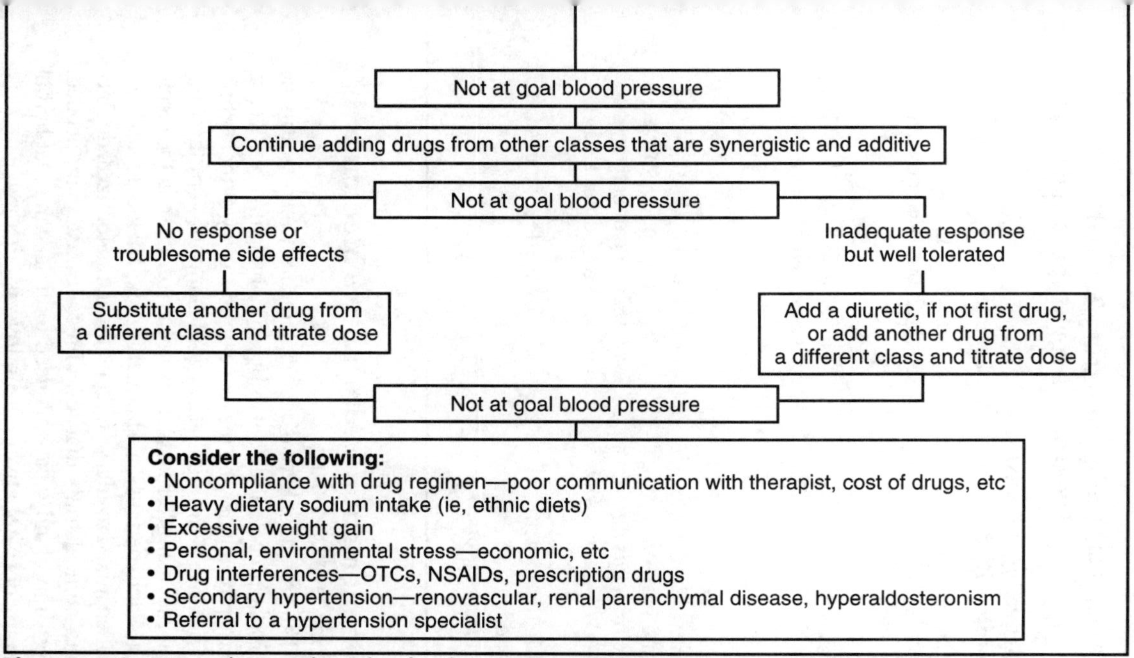

Figure 6-3: Compilation algorithm for the treatment of hypertension in African Americans.

Table 6-4: Complementary/Herbal Treatments for Hypertension

Active ingredients/ preparation	Dosage
Garlic cloves	4 g fresh garlic cloves or 600-1,200 g dried powder
Rauwolfia root	Maintenance dose 50-300 mg of powdered whole root
Hawthorn leaves and blossom (*Crataegus monogyna* and *Crataegus laevigata*)	1 g herb daily Instructions: pour hot water over 0.2-0.3 g of herb and infuse, 3 to 4 times a day
Mistletoe stem and leaves (*Viscum album*)	No known effective dosage

Complementary/Alternative Medicine in Hypertension

The growth of herbal or complementary medicine in the pharmaceutical industry has been dramatic in recent years. Many physicians who make a careful survey of their clinical practice will find that a significant portion of their patients are using herbal therapy or have done so in the recent past. For hypertension, alternative or herbal medicines have yielded mixed results so far, but larger, randomized, double-blind clinical trials that test clinical efficacy are needed. Most importantly, patients need to understand that herbal therapy does not always mean low-risk therapy.

Comments

Potentially useful for mild stage 1 hypertension. Risks: may cause gastrointestinal complaints, bleeding, especially if on warfarin.

May be helpful in treating mild essential hypertension; may be especially useful in anxiety-associated hypertension. Risks: may cause depression, fatigue, and problems with sexual potency.

May be of some use as a supportive treatment for blood pressure lowering. Risks: may cause nausea, headache, vertigo; may increase digoxin toxicity.

Not effective against high blood pressure.

Garlic

Garlic has probably received the most attention as a treatment for hypertension (Table 6-4). It has been touted by some authors as a mild antihypertensive, a lipid-lowering agent, and an antioxidant. Under ideal circumstances, garlic can only be considered as a potential treatment for mild (stage 1) hypertension. Adverse effects such as nausea, vomiting, and diarrhea have been reported, but it is the potential risk of bleeding that raises the most concern. At least one report cited a spontaneous spinal epidermal, and other reports have shown increased prothrombin times in patients taking garlic. In summary, garlic appears to have modest lipid-lowering and antihypertensive properties but should probably not be used by patients taking warfarin and antiplatelet agents. One recent Yale University study found that garlic failed to cause any significant decrease in blood pressure and cholesterol versus placebo. At this point, it seems safe to say that more research is needed before the FDA approves garlic therapy as effective hypertension management.

Acupuncture

Acupuncture is frequently used to treat hypertension in Asia and in some parts of the West. In one small, uncontrolled study of 50 patients with untreated essential hypertension, patients were given a 30-minute acupuncture treatment that resulted in a significant reduction in blood pressure and heart rate. The practitioners of acupuncture believe that blood pressure reduction is a result of an endocrine mechanism, and in fact, in this study, a significant decline occurred in plasma renin activity. Interestingly, there was no significant change in serum cortisol levels or vasopressin levels. Obviously, larger controlled clinical trials are needed.

Ginseng

Ginseng is a popular herbal remedy for a variety of ailments, but it has been reported to increase blood pressure.

Most herbal remedies on the market have not been tested extensively with other pharmacologic agents, so clinicians often do not have adequate data to properly counsel patients on potential drug interactions. While some herbal remedies probably will eventually receive FDA approval, clinicians should be cautious about using them until more extensive efficacy trials have been completed.

Selected Readings

ABC Digest of Urban Cardiology 1997;4:12.

Brenner BM, Cooper ME, de Zeeuw D et al: Effects of losartan on renal and cardiovascular outcomes in patients with type 2 diabetes and nephropathy. *N Engl J Med* 2001;345:861-869.

Dahlof B, Devereux RB, Kjeldsen SE, et al: Cardiovascular morbidity and mortality in the Losartan Intervention for Endpoint reduction in hypertension study (LIFE): a randomised trial against atenolol. *Lancet* 2002;359:995-1003.

Douglas JG, Bakris GL, Epstein M, et al: Management of high blood pressure in African Americans: consensus statement of the Hypertension in African Americans Working Group of the International Society on Hypertension in Blacks. *Arch Intern Med* 2003;163:525-541.

Elliott WJ: Higher incidence of discontinuation of angiotensin converting enzyme inhibitors due to cough in black subjects. *Clin Pharmacol Ther* 1996;60:582-588.

Flack JM: Reducing the CV risk burden: the role of AII blockade. Cardiovascular Summit Highlights. May 2002; 11-14.

Goldberg AI, Dunlay MC, Sweet CS: Safety and tolerability of losartan potassium, an angiotensin II receptor antagonist, compared with hydrochlorothiazide, atenolol, felodipine ER, and angiotensin-converting enzyme inhibitors for the treatment of systemic hypertension. *Am J Cardiol* 1995;75:793-795.

Johnson WR, Saunders E: Management of high risk hypertensive patients. *Cardiology Special Edition* 2002;8:15-21.

Isaacsohn JL, Moser M, Stein EA, et al: Garlic powder and plasma lipids and lipoproteins: a multicenter, randomized, placebo-controlled trial. *Arch Intern Med* 1998;158:1189-1194.

Lewis EJ, Hunsicker LG, Clarke WR, et al: Renoprotective effect of the angiotensin-receptor antagonist irbesartan in patients with nephropathy due to type 2 diabetes. *N Engl J Med* 2001;345:851-860.

Major outcomes in high-risk hypertensive patients randomized to angiotensin-converting enzyme inhibitor or calcium channel blocker vs diuretic: The Antihypertensive and Lipid-Lowering Treatment to Prevent Heart Attack Trial (ALLHAT). *JAMA* 2002; 288:2981-2997.

Materson BJ, Reda DJ, Cushman WC, et al: Single-drug therapy for hypertension in men. A comparison of six antihypertensive agents with placebo. The Department of Veteran Affairs Cooperative Study Group on Antihypertensive Agents. *N Engl J Med* 1993; 328:914-921.

Micozzi MS: *Current Review of Complementary Medicine.* Philadelphia: Current Medicine Inc, 1999, pp 1-167.

Moser M, Hebert PR: Prevention of disease progression, left ventricular hypertrophy and congestive heart failure in hypertension treatment trials. *J Am Coll Cardiol* 1996;27:1214-1218.

Oparil S, Williams D, Chrysant SG, et al: Comparative efficacy of olmesartan, losartan, valsartan, and irbesartan in the control of essential hypertension. *J Clin Hypertens (Greenwich)* 2001;3:283-291, 318.

Parving HH, Lehnert H, Brochner-Mortensen J, et al: The effect of irbesartan on the development of diabetic nephropathy in patients with type 2 diabetes. *N Engl J Med* 2001;345:870-878.

Psaty BM, Smith NL, Siscovick DS, et al: Health outcomes associated with antihypertensive therapies used as first-line agents. A systematic review and meta-analysis. *JAMA* 1997;277:739-745.

Ram CV: Pharmacologic differences among calcium channel blockers: basis for rational therapy decisions. *Preventive Cardiology Clinic (Suppl Cardiology Review)* 2002:3-6.

Sareli P, Radevski IV, Valtchanova ZP, et al: Efficacy of different drug classes used to initiate antihypertensive treatment in black subjects: results of a randomized trial in Johannesburg, South Africa. *Arch Intern Med* 2001;161:965-971.

Saunders E: A new paradigm for management of high-risk hypertensive patients. Presented at the American Society of Hypertension. May 20, 1999. Abstract.

Saunders E, Gavin JR 3rd: Blockade of the renin-angiotensin system in African-Americans with hypertension and cardiovascular disease. *J Clin Hypertens (Greenwich)* 2003;5(suppl 1):12-17.

Saunders E, Weir MR, Kong BW, et al: A comparison of the efficacy and safety of a β-blocker, a calcium-channel blocker, and a converting enzyme inhibitor in hypertensive blacks. *Arch Intern Med* 1990;150:1707-1713.

The Seventh Report of the Joint National Committee on Prevention, Detection, Evaluation, and Treatment of High Blood Pressure. *JAMA* 2003;289:2560-2572.

Treatment of hypertension in adults with diabetes (position statement). *Diabetes Care* 2003;26(suppl 1):S80-S82.

Weber MA: Angiotensin II receptor blockers. *Cardiology Special Edition* 2002;8:38-42.

Wright JT Jr, Bakris G, Greene T, et al: Effect of blood pressure lowering and antihypertension drug class on progression of hypertensive kidney disease: results from the AASK Trial. *JAMA* 2002;288:2421-2431.

Zanchetti A: Efficacy and tolerability of lercanidipine in elderly hypertensives: results of a multicenter, double-blind, randomized study. *Am J Hypertens* 2002;15(4 Suppl 1);A117.

Chapter 7

Role of Community Programs in the Management of Hypertension in African Americans

The medical profession has recognized the importance of forming partnerships with churches, synagogues, and other community organizations to help promote better health care. The appropriate treatment and control of hypertension in African-American communities can occur only with a population-wide strategy to detect and prevent high blood pressure. An effective way to reach this population is to establish a relationship with the institutions that reflect a community's beliefs and values. Essentially, we are talking about large-scale behavior modification.

The first step to any community-based program for African Americans is to gain support for the program from organizations such as churches, schools, social clubs, and even neighborhood barbershops. These groups can then participate in an intensive education program on hypertension and other cardiovascular diseases. As reported by Saunders et al in 1991, these programs can be more far-reaching if they are first held in churches, which serve as centers for most community education programs for blacks. Community churches can conceivably serve as places where African Americans can be educated about guidelines on appropriate diet, weight control, blood pressure control, exercise, smoking cessation, and substance abuse.

Once the concept of education programs is accepted by churches or other organizations, the next step is to identify designated leaders who can help to conduct a definitive, organized curriculum. In Baltimore, Maryland, community health organizations, such as the Baltimore Alliance, Church CHAMP, and the Mind, Heart, and Body Program, work with churches to develop education programs and schedule workshops and health fairs to educate congregations. One goal, over time, is to train some members of the congregation to take blood pressures regularly and do dietary and weight control counseling. These measures would promote better blood pressure control once the goal blood pressure is achieved.

This model could then be used in other organizations such as fraternities, sororities, lodges, and social clubs.

Even some neighborhood barbershops have adopted blood pressure screening programs based on the church model. But these have been more difficult to establish and maintain, probably because of the need for more training and monitoring of activities.

In addition, dentists, pharmacists, podiatrists, nutritionists, community health nurses, and many other health care professionals can be trained to screen and monitor blood pressures.

Selected Readings

Pearson TA, Jenkins GM, Thomas J: Prevention of coronary heart disease in black adults. In: Saunders E, ed. *Cardiovascular Diseases in Blacks*. Philadelphia, FA Davis, 1991, p 272.

Saunders E, ed: *Cardiovascular Diseases in Blacks*. Philadelphia, FA Davis, 1991, p 342.

Chapter 8

Prevention of Hypertension

The process of primary prevention of hypertension through lifestyle modification has been addressed in Chapter 6. In this chapter, we want to go a step further by advocating that the private and public sectors become involved in community and corporate initiatives to significantly reduce the incidence of hypertension in African Americans.

For example, industries whose products can adversely affect the African-American community (such as tobacco and fast-food companies) should join this effort. The tobacco industry has already been ordered to pay billions of dollars to various state treasuries because costly treatments for smoke-induced illnesses previously were largely paid for with state revenues.

Large industries can support community outreach groups that strive to improve the health of citizens. The industries would benefit by having a healthier, more educated workforce.

We believe that the fast-food and supermarket industries should work to provide lower-fat, low-salt alternatives of popular African-American staples at reasonable prices. Innovative nutritionists can learn how to 'soulize' food without excessive sodium, fat, or cholesterol content. Employers should be encouraged to provide exercise facilities or to strongly support use of such facilities near job sites. Employers should also invite community health organizations to conduct workshops and health fairs whenever possible.

Another important part of preventing hypertension is the prevention of target organ damage in patients with diagnosed hypertension. Again, partnerships are a key component because noncompliance is a major cause of hypertension-induced target organ damage. Community organizations that partner with clinicians can do a great deal to increase compliance. Pharmacists are also good sources of information on medical compliance and often have a marked influence on patient education and behavior. By working as a team, medical professionals and public and private organizations can make significant progress in preventing hypertension in African Americans.

Conclusion

We do not know definitively why hypertension is such a major problem in African Americans and people of African descent who assume a Western lifestyle. An interaction of a certain predisposition (possibly genetic) with environmental factors (eg, psychosocial factors, diet) is likely responsible. No single factor appears to be sufficient to produce this widespread and serious problem, with its numerous cardiovascular complications (eg, heart, renal, cerebrovascular), among African Americans. Research into the etiology and pathophysiology of, and treatment strategies for, hypertension continues, but much more is needed. We are gratified that the National Heart, Lung, and Blood Institute is increasingly involved in studies (ALLHAT and AASK) that will help to answer many questions about hypertension treatment, especially for African Americans. Importantly, these two studies, supported by the National Institutes of Health, have already begun to affect how we manage hypertensive patients, especially African Americans with renal disease, as is seen in the recently completed AASK study. With rapidly developing research in vascular biology, we will probably see other changes in the near future. Credit should be extended to the pharmaceutical industry, which has sponsored numerous studies, often with intermediate end points, but some with long-term outcomes, that have helped significantly in altering our treatment strategies. Studies such as TREND, TRACE, HOT, HOPE, IDNT, IRMA-2, RENAAL, and VAL-HeFT, to name some, have confirmed the importance of lowering blood pressure. These studies have suggested other benefits, especially in high-risk populations such as diabetic patients and the elderly, with the use of angiotensin-converting enzyme inhibitors, angiotensin-receptor blockers, calcium-channel blockers, diuretics, and combinations of many of these agents to achieve better outcomes. New studies such as PEACE, AVALON, PROGRESS, CONQUER, and VALUE are under way or were recently completed.

As indicated throughout this book, we believe that African Americans represent a high-risk population for hypertension that is often undiagnosed or diagnosed only after target organ damage has occurred. Thus, treatment is often inadequate and/or inappropriate. Although much of this is related to poor patient compliance and adherence, the professional and nonprofessional communities must bear some responsibility. Physicians treating these patients need to be familiar with many of the issues addressed in this book. We recognize that most physicians are not African Americans and therefore may need to make a special effort to learn about some of the unique aspects of African-American culture. They also need to be culturally competent and try to understand some of the practices of African Americans that may have a bearing on blood pressure and treatment. Many physicians practicing in urban areas are non-African-American minorities, which may present not only cultural disparity, but also language barriers.

Economic issues and lack of access to medical care are problems in African-American communities that have a major impact on outcomes in hypertensive blacks. The low physician/patient ratio and inconvenient office hours and locations in African-American neighborhoods are also problems.

Finally, we hope that local and regional government agencies, as well as the private sector, will recognize that no society is more healthy than its most unhealthy component. Therefore, it remains the responsibility of the entire community to deal with the problem of hypertension in African Americans, not only because of economic costs, but also because of the lost productivity of a large part of our society and the high rate of disability and premature death resulting from this disease.

Appendix

Selected Guidelines of the JNC 7 Report

Table 1: Cardiovascular Risk Factors

Major Risk Factors

- Hypertension*
- Cigarette smoking
- Obesity (BMI ≥30)*
- Physical inactivity
- Dyslipidemia*
- Diabetes mellitus*
- Microalbuminuria or estimated GFR <60 mL/min
- Age (>55 years for men, >65 years for women)
- Family history of premature cardiovascular disease (men <55 years or women <65 years)

(continued on next page)

BMI = body mass index (weight [kg] divided by height [m^2])

GFR = glomerular filtration rate

*Components of the metabolic syndrome

National Heart, Lung, and Blood Institute: *JNC 7 Express: The Seventh Report of the Joint National Committee on Prevention, Detection, Evaluation, and Treatment of High Blood Pressure.* Rockville, MD, US Department of Health and Human Services; May 2003. NIH Publication no. 03-5233.

Table 1: Cardiovascular Risk Factors *(continued)*

Target Organ Damage

- Heart
  - Left ventricular hypertrophy
  - Angina or prior myocardial infarction
  - Prior coronary revascularization
  - Heart failure
- Brain
  - Stroke or transient ischemic attack
- Chronic kidney disease
- Peripheral arterial disease
- Retinopathy

National Heart, Lung, and Blood Institute: *JNC 7 Express: The Seventh Report of the Joint National Committee on Prevention, Detection, Evaluation, and Treatment of High Blood Pressure.* Rockville, MD, US Department of Health and Human Services; May 2003. NIH Publication no. 03-5233.

Table 2: Identifiable Causes of Hypertension

- Sleep apnea
- Drug-induced or drug-related causes
  - Nonadherence
  - Inadequate doses
  - Inappropriate combinations
  - Nonsteroidal anti-inflammatory drugs; cyclooxygenase 2 inhibitors
  - Cocaine, amphetamines, other illicit drugs
  - Sympathomimetics (decongestants, anorectics)
  - Oral contraceptives
  - Adrenal steroids
  - Cyclosporine and tacrolimus
  - Erythropoietin
  - Licorice (including some chewing tobacco)
  - Selected over-the-counter dietary supplements and medicines (eg, ephedra, ma huang, bitter orange)
- Chronic kidney disease
- Primary aldosteronism
- Renovascular disease
- Chronic steroid therapy and Cushing's syndrome
- Pheochromocytoma
- Coarctation of the aorta
- Thyroid or parathyroid disease

National Heart, Lung, and Blood Institute: *JNC 7 Express: The Seventh Report of the Joint National Committee on Prevention, Detection, Evaluation, and Treatment of High Blood Pressure.* Rockville, MD, US Department of Health and Human Services; May 2003. NIH Publication no. 03-5233.

Table 3: Clinical Trial and Guideline Basis for Compelling Indications for Individual Drug Classes

Compelling Indication*
Heart failure
Post-myocardial infarction
High coronary disease risk
Diabetes
Chronic kidney disease
Recurrent stroke prevention

* Compelling indications for antihypertensive drugs are based on benefits from outcome studies or existing clinical guidelines; the compelling indication is managed in parallel with the blood pressure.

** Conditions for which clinical trials demonstrate benefit of specific classes of antihypertensive drugs

BB = β-blocker; ACEI = angiotensin-converting enzyme

Recommended Drugs

Diuretic	BB	ACEI	ARB	CCB	Aldo ANT	Clinical Trial Basis**
•	•	•	•		•	ACC/AHA Heart Failure Guideline, MERIT-HF, COPERNICUS, CIBIS, SOLVD, AIRE, TRACE, ValHEFT, RALES
	•	•			•	ACC/AHA Post-MI Guideline, BHAT, SAVE, CAPRICORN, EPHESUS
•	•	•		•		ALLHAT, HOPE, ANBP2, LIFE, CONVINCE
•	•	•	•	•		NKF-ADA Guideline, UKPDS, ALLHAT
		•	•			NKF Guideline, Captopril Trial, RENAAL, IDNT, REIN, AASK
•		•				PROGRESS

inhibitor; ARB = angiotensin II receptor blocker; CCB = calcium-channel blocker; Aldo ANT = aldosterone antagonist

National Heart, Lung, and Blood Institute: *JNC 7 Express: The Seventh Report of the Joint National Committee on Prevention, Detection, Evaluation, and Treatment of High Blood Pressure.* Rockville, MD, US Department of Health and Human Services; May 2003. NIH Publication no. 03-5233.

Index

A

α-agonists 57
α-β-blockers 76, 105, 133
α-blockers 43, 92, 105, 125, 133
α-receptor blockers 36, 57
abdominal bloating 31
Accupril® 122
Aceon® 100
Actos® 27
acupuncture 136
Adalat® 124
adrenergic agents 28
adrenergic blockers 129
adrenergic/serotoninergic agents 28
aerobic activity 36, 133
aerobics 30
African Americans 8, 9, 11, 16, 21, 22, 24, 30, 32, 33, 37, 41, 43, 48, 49, 58, 60, 64, 76, 77, 85-87, 91-93, 95, 98, 99, 104, 111, 116, 117, 122, 126, 127, 129, 133, 139, 141-144
African-American Study of Kidney Disease and Hypertension (AASK) 95, 98, 99, 125, 128, 129, 142
alcohol 32, 34, 36, 67, 73, 74, 108, 118, 133
almonds 63
Altace® 40, 96, 122
American Diabetes Association 36, 43, 104, 105
American Heart Association 24
American Society of Hypertension (ASH) 45, 114
amlodipine (Norvasc®) 35, 37, 42, 96, 97, 102, 103, 125, 128, 130
amphetamines 75
amputations 42
anesthesia 30
angina pectoris 30, 146
angiotensin-converting enzyme (ACE) inhibitors 7, 35-37, 39, 40, 41, 43, 48, 56, 57, 64, 65, 86, 92, 96, 98-100, 102, 104, 105, 121, 122, 124, 128, 129, 131, 133, 148, 149
angiotensin-receptor blockers (ARBs) 7, 35, 42, 86, 99, 102-105, 121, 122, 124, 128-131, 133, 149
Antihypertensive and Lipid Lowering Treatment to Prevent Heart Attack Trial (ALLHAT) 125, 127, 142
antiobesity agents 30, 33
antioxidant 135
anxiety 112, 135
aortic aneurysm 90, 92
apnea 32
appetite control 24

appetite suppressants 28
Appropriate Blood Pressure Control in Diabetes (ABCD) trials 35
Apresoline® 43
apricots 63, 66
arterial occlusive disease 93
arteriography 111
artichokes 63
asparagus 66
aspirin 41, 94
atenolol (Tenormin®) 38, 124, 127, 128, 131
atherosclerosis 49, 120, 128
atherosclerotic disease 90, 94
AVALON 143
Avandia® 27
Avapro® 35, 102, 130
avocado 66

B

β-3 agonists 28
β-blockers 7, 37-39, 41-43, 50, 57, 65, 76, 86, 96, 97, 105, 121, 122, 128, 130, 148, 149
bagels 63
bananas 63, 64, 66
barbershops 139, 140
beans 63, 66
beer 73
behavior modification 29, 60, 139
benzphetamine 28
bile acid sequestrates 56
bleeding 135
blindness 90
blood pressure 7, 9, 11, 16, 17, 20, 21, 25, 30, 32, 33, 35-39, 41, 43, 50, 58, 60, 61, 64, 65, 67, 73, 75-78, 85, 86, 90-92, 95-97, 100, 107, 109-114, 116, 117, 122, 125, 128, 129, 133, 136, 139
measurement 108
body mass index (BMI) 26, 46, 118, 145
brain ischemia 92
bread 60, 62, 63
broccoli 63, 66
bruits 111
bupropion (Wellbutrin®, Zyban®) 30, 70, 71
butter 60
buttermilk 63

C

caffeine 28, 60, 108, 112, 113
calcium 22, 48, 63-65, 133
calcium antagonists 7, 36, 57, 65, 133
calcium-channel blockers 35, 41, 43, 76, 86, 96, 97, 105, 121, 122, 124, 129, 130, 149
cantaloupe 66
Capoten® 38, 124
captopril (Capoten®) 38, 124, 127
Captopril Prevention Project (CAPP) 37, 38
cardiac arrhythmias 73, 74
cardiac disease 49
Cardizem® 124
cardiovascular disease (CVD) 7, 11, 30, 31, 40, 67, 85, 108, 125, 145

cardiovascular morbidity 117
cardiovascular mortality 40, 48, 103
Cardura® 125
carotid artery stenosis 92, 94
carrots 63, 66
Cartia XT® 124
carvedilol (Coreg®) 56
Catapres® 124
catecholamines 32, 74, 110
cereals 62, 63
cerebral aneurysm 92
cerebrovascular disease 91-93, 110
cheese 62
chest pain 44
chlorthalidone (Hygroton®, Thalitone®) 37, 125
cholesterol 39, 49, 50, 64, 94, 110, 133, 136, 141
  high-density lipoprotein (HDL) cholesterol 45, 49-51, 110
  low-density lipoprotein (LDL) cholesterol 44, 50, 51, 56, 57
cigarette smoking 67, 71, 90, 145
cigars 67
clonidine (Catapres®) 124
cocaine 73-75, 147
cold pressor test 21
collards 63
community organizations 140
community programs 14, 139, 141
complementary/alternative medicine 134
compliance 143
Consequences of the Reversal of Endothelial Dysfunction With Use of Quinapril (CONQUER Study) 121, 128, 143
continuous positive airway pressure (CPAP) 32
Coreg® 56
coronary artery disease (CAD) 24, 31, 39, 46, 49, 87
coronary heart disease (CHD) 13, 37, 44, 49, 51, 85, 87, 94
corticosteroid 45
cortisol 136
Cozaar® 35, 102, 130
Crataegus laevigata 134
Crataegus monogyna 134
creatinine 100, 110

D

dairy products 59
dates 63, 66
depression 30, 135
dexfenfluramine 28
diabetes 7, 33, 34, 37, 39, 40, 42, 43, 46, 48, 50, 87, 90, 102, 104, 105, 110, 120, 129, 131, 133, 145, 148
  type 1 34
  type 2 26, 34, 35, 37, 41, 46, 47
diabetic retinopathy 34
dialysis 95
diarrhea 135
diet 29, 30, 58, 140
Dietary Approaches to Stop Hypertension (DASH) diet 22, 59, 61-63, 116, 118

dietary counseling 60
dietary modifications 58, 60
diethylpropion 28
digestive inhibitors 29
digoxin 135
dihydropyridines 124
Dilacor XR® 124
Diltia XT® 124
diltiazem (Cardizem®, Cartia XT®, Dilacor XR®, Diltia XT®, Tiazac®) 124
Diovan® 65, 103
diuretics 7, 36-39, 50, 57, 61, 86, 96, 105, 121, 122, 125, 129-131, 133, 149
dizziness 91
dopamine 74
dopamine β-hydroxylase 21
doxazosin (Cardura®) 125
dyslipidemia 26, 27, 36, 40, 45, 47-49, 90, 110, 145
dysmetabolic syndrome 45

E

echocardiogram 86
echocardiography 110
eclampsia 60
economic discrimination 76
edema 111, 125
Effexor® 30
electrocardiogram 85
electrolyte disturbances 122
end-stage renal disease (ESRD) 11, 34, 95, 126, 131
endarterectomy 94
endothelial dysfunction 120, 128
endothelin 21, 74
endotheliopathy 128
environmental factors 16
ephedrine 28
Esidrix® 37, 122
ethanol 112
exercise 29, 30, 33, 42, 60, 72, 140, 141

F

fat consumption 31, 59
fat substitutes 29
fatigue 135
felodipine (Plendil®) 39, 125
fenfluramine 28
fiber 61, 63
fibric acid derivatives 56
fibrinolysis 45
filberts 63
fish 62
flatulence 31
fluoxetine 28
Food and Drug Administration (FDA) 29, 124, 136
Fosinopril Versus Amlodipine Cardiovascular Events (FACET) trial 35
Framingham Heart Study 25, 50, 52, 54, 85
Framingham Point Scores 52-55
fruits 61, 62
furosemide 20

G

garlic 60, 134, 135
gastrointestinal complaints 135
gemfibrozil (Lopid®) 56
genetic aberrations 16

ginseng 136
glitazones 27, 48
Glucophage® 27
glucose 26, 43-46, 51, 110
glucose intolerance 45
goal blood pressure 34, 43, 94, 95, 129, 133, 140
gout 46, 110
grains 62
grapefruit 66
grapes 63
grits 63
growth receptors 21

H

Habitrol® 67, 68
hawthorn leaves 134
headache 91, 135
health insurance 77
heart disease 9
heart failure 7, 90, 133, 146, 148
Heart Outcomes Prevention Evaluation (HOPE) Study 39, 40, 48, 99, 122, 129, 143
herbal remedies 108, 134, 136
hormonal manipulation 29
hydralazine (Apresoline®) 43, 56, 57
hydrochlorothiazide (Esidrix®, HydroDIURIL®, Microzide®, Oretic®) 37, 122
HydroDIURIL® 37, 122
Hygroton® 37, 125
hyperaldosteronism 133
hypercapnia 32
hyperglycemia 36
hyperinsulinemia 47
hyperlipidemia 47
hypertension 6, 7, 9, 11, 14, 16, 19, 21, 25, 27, 30-32, 34, 39, 40, 43, 45, 47-49, 58, 61, 64, 65, 74, 75, 77, 78, 87, 91-95, 102-105, 107, 109-111, 114, 116, 117, 120, 122, 129, 133-135, 139, 141-145
Hypertension Optimal Treatment (HOT) trial 38, 143
hypertension specialists 45, 114
hypertriglyceridemia 46
hyperuricemia 46
hypoxemia 32

I

illicit drug use 108
impaired hearing 112
indapamide (Lozol®) 100, 101
insulin 22, 26, 27, 44, 45, 47
insulin resistance 21, 22, 44-48
insulin resistance syndrome 26, 44
International Society on Hypertension in Blacks 8, 116, 121, 129
intracranial artery occlusive disease 92, 93
intracranial hemorrhage 92
irbesartan (Avapro®) 35, 42, 102, 103, 130
Irbesartan Diabetic Nephropathy Trial (IDNT) 35, 43, 102, 130

Irbesartan Microalbuminuria Type 2 Diabetes in Hypertensive Patients Study (IRMA-2) 35, 42, 103, 130
ischemic heart disease 87, 88

J

J-curve 38
Joint National Committee on Prevention, Detection, Evaluation and Treatment of High Blood Pressure 14, 43, 116
Seventh Report (JNC 7) 6, 7, 34, 59, 61, 73, 94, 102, 107, 114, 116, 122, 128, 145
Sixth Report (JNC 6) 6, 7, 110

K

Kaiser-Permanente Multiphasic Health Examination Study 72
kale 63
kallikrein 21
kidney beans 63
kidney failure 42, 96
Korotkoff phase I 109

L

labetalol (Normodyne®, Trandate®) 56, 76, 92
lacidipine 125
leaky bulb valve 112
left ventricular dysfunction 129
left ventricular hypertrophy (LVH) 74, 75, 85, 86, 146
legumes 62
lentils 63
leptin analogs 29
lercanidipine 124, 125
lifestyle modifications 36, 49-51, 60, 116-118, 121, 133
lipase inhibitors 29
lipases 31
lipid abnormalities 49
lipid-lowering therapy 41, 56, 135
lipids 26, 43-45, 49, 57, 94
Loniten® 43
loose stools 31
Lopid® 56
Lopressor® 97
losartan (Cozaar®) 35, 43, 102, 103, 130, 131
Losartan Intervention for Endpoint Reduction in Hypertension (LIFE) study 86, 131
loss of balance 91
Lozol® 100

M

magnesium 22, 60, 63, 65, 133
magnetic resonance angiography (MRA) 92, 111
mangoes 63
manometer 108, 112
marijuana 75
mazindol 28
meats 62, 63
medical history 109
melons 63
mental illness 75

mercury 112
Meridia® 30
metformin (Glucophage®) 27, 48
metoprolol (Lopressor®, Toprol XL®) 97
microalbuminuria 6, 35, 40, 102-104, 130, 133, 145
Microalbuminuria Reduction with Valsartan (MARVAL) trial 103
Microzide® 37, 122
milk 62, 63
minerals 61
Minipress® 124
minoxidil (Loniten®) 43, 56, 57
mistletoe stem 134
Modification of Diet in Renal Disease (MDRD) study 95
mozzarella cheese 63
muffins 63
Multiple Risk Factor Intervention Trial (MRFIT) 49
murmurs 111
mushrooms 66
myocardial infarction (MI) 38, 40, 74, 86, 88, 92, 94, 131, 133, 146, 148

N

National Cholesterol Education Program (NCEP) 49-51, 94
National Health and Examination Survey 49
National Health and Nutrition Examination Survey III (NHANES III) 24, 34
National Heart, Lung, and Blood Institute (NHLBI) 65, 142
National Institutes of Health (NIH) 33, 95, 142
National Kidney Foundation 36
National Stroke Association 94
natriuretic peptides 21
nausea 135
nefazodone (Serzone®) 30
nephropathy 35, 37, 41, 42, 102-104, 128, 130
nephrosclerosis 95
Nicoderm CQ® 67, 68
Nicorette® 70
nicotine 67
nicotine patches 67, 72
nicotinic acid 56
Nicotrol® 67, 68, 70
nifedipine (Adalat®, Procardia®) 124
nisoldipine (Sular®) 37
nitric oxide 49
nitroglycerin 76
Nitropress® 76, 92
nitroprusside (Nitropress®) 76, 92
nitrous oxide 74
nocturnal blood pressures 21
nonadrenergic agents 28
noncompliance 133
nonfat dairy foods 62
nonsteroidal anti-inflammatory drugs (NSAIDs) 133, 147
norepinephrine 21
Normodyne® 56, 92

Norvasc® 35, 96, 125
numbness 91
nuts 62

O

oatmeal 63
obesity 6, 24-28, 32-34, 46, 47, 87, 116, 145
olestra 29
optic fundi 90
oral glucose tolerance test (OGTT) 46
orange juice 63, 66
oranges 63, 66
Oretic® 37, 122
organomegaly 111
orlistat (Xenical®) 29-31
osteoporosis 64
ouabain-like sodium pump inhibitor 21

P

pain 112
parallax error 112
pasta 62
PEACE 143
peaches 63, 66
peanuts 63, 66
peas 63
perindopril (Aceon®) 100, 101
Perindopril Protection Against Recurrent Stroke Study (PROGRESS) 100, 101
peripheral vascular disease (PVD) 39, 40, 90, 110
pharmacists 142
phendimetrazine 28
phentermine 28, 30, 31
phenylephrine 113
physical examination 110, 111
pickwickian syndrome 32
pineapples 63
pioglitazone (Actos®) 27, 48
pita bread 63
plasma renin activity (PRA) 20
Plendil® 39, 125
polycystic ovary syndrome 45
polysomnography 31
potassium 21, 25, 56, 63-66, 110, 133
potatoes 63, 66
poultry 62, 63
prazosin (Minipress®) 124
premature death 87
probucol 56
Procardia® 124
prostaglandin 21
ProStep® 67
protein 60, 63
proteinuria 35, 36, 44, 96, 133
prunes 63, 66
psychosocial issues 76, 109
pulmonary edema 92

Q

quinapril (Accupril®) 122

R

race 11, 16
racism 76
raisins 63, 66
rales 111
ramipril (Altace®) 40, 41, 96, 97, 122, 128

rauwolfia root 134
Reductil® 30
Reduction of Endpoints in NIDDM with the Angiotensin II Antagonist Losartan (RENAAL) study 35, 43, 102, 130, 143
religion and medicine 78
religious faith 77
renal disease 41, 43, 95, 102, 105, 110, 117, 133, 142
renal failure 75
renal insufficiency 95
renal scan 111
renin 110, 122
renin hypersensitivity 21
renin-angiotensin-aldosterone system (RAAS) 16, 17, 128
reserpine 57
retinopathy 90, 111, 146
rhonchi 111
rice 62
rosiglitazone (Avandia®) 27, 48

S

saline 20
salt 61, 64, 65, 73, 122, 141
seeds 62
serotonin 74
serotoninergic agents 28
sertraline 28
Serzone® 30
sexual dysfunction 110
sexual potency 135
shock 93, 112
sibutramine (Meridia®, Reductil®) 28, 30, 31
sleep apnea 6, 31, 32, 147
sleep disordered breathing (SDB) 31
sleepiness 33
smoking 32, 36, 40, 78, 112
smoking cessation 67, 140
snoring 33
socioeconomic factors 76, 109, 117
sodium 18, 19, 21, 25-27, 34, 36, 47, 58-61, 64-66, 74, 108, 110, 124, 133, 141
sodium-channel blocker 74
somnolence 32
sphygmomanometer 108, 111
spinach 63, 66
squash 63, 66
starch 61
statin drugs 56, 94
stethoscope 108, 112
strawberries 63
stress 77, 133
stroke 9, 12, 22, 30, 37, 39, 40, 73, 74, 85, 86, 91-93, 100, 112, 117, 120, 131, 146, 148
substance abuse 67, 75, 140
Sular® 37
sunflower seeds 63, 66
sweet potatoes 63, 66
Systolic Hypertension in the Elderly Program (SHEP) 37

T

tachycardia 76
tangerines 63

target organ damage 9, 11, 16, 21, 74, 85, 110, 114, 117, 128, 142, 143, 146
Tenormin® 38, 124
tetrahydrocannabinol (THC) 75
Thalitone® 37, 125
thermogenic agents 28
Third Report of the National Cholesterol Education Program Expert Panel on Detection, Evaluation, and Treatment of High Blood Cholesterol in Adults 51
thrombolytic therapy 92
thyroid 111
thyroid disease 30
thyroid stimulating hormone 110
Tiazac® 124
tissue plasminogen activator (TPA) 92
tobacco 67, 108, 133, 141
tomatoes 63, 66
Toprol XL® 97
TRACE 143
Trandate® 56, 92
transcranial Doppler (TCD) 92
transient ischemic attack (TIA) 39, 100, 146
TREND 143
triglycerides 44, 45, 49-51, 56, 57
turnip greens 63

U

U.S. Renal Data System 95, 96
ultrasound 92, 111
unemployment 77
United Kingdom Prospective Diabetes Study (UKPDS) 37

V

valsartan (Diovan®) 65, 103
Valsartan Heart Failure Trial (ValHeFT) 87
vascular dementia 93
vascular disease 111
vascular endothelial dysfunction 48
vascular hypertrophy 26, 47
vascular resistance 20
vasoconstrictor receptors 21
vasodilators 43, 129
vasopressin levels 136
vegetables 61, 62
venlafaxine (Effexor®) 30
verapamil (Calan®, Covera®, Isoptin®, Verelan®) 127
vertigo 135
Viscum album 134
visual impairment 42
Vital Statistics of the United States, National Center for Health Statistics 11-13
vitamin E 41
vitamins 61
vomiting 135

W

waist-to-hip ratio 45
walking clubs 30
walnuts 63
warfarin 135, 136
watermelon 66
weakness 91

weight control 42, 51, 140
weight gain 25, 72, 133
weight loss 24, 25, 28, 30, 33, 34, 36, 58, 60, 64, 119, 133
Wellbutrin® 30
wheezes 111
white coat hypertension 112, 114
wine 73

X

Xenical® 30

Y

'yo-yo' dieting 33
yogurt 62, 63

Z

Zyban® 30, 70, 71

Rx only

AVAPRO®
(irbesartan) Tablets
AVALIDE®
(irbesartan-hydrochlorothiazide) Tablets

USE IN PREGNANCY

When used in pregnancy during the second and third trimesters, drugs that act directly on the renin-angiotensin system can cause injury and even death to the developing fetus. When pregnancy is detected, AVAPRO and AVALIDE should be discontinued as soon as possible. (See **WARNINGS: Fetal/Neonatal Morbidity and Mortality**.)

DESCRIPTION

AVAPRO®* (irbesartan) is an angiotensin II receptor (AT_1 subtype) antagonist. AVALIDE®* (irbesartan-hydrochlorothiazide) Tablets is a combination of an angiotensin II receptor antagonist (AT_1 subtype), irbesartan, and a thiazide diuretic, hydrochlorothiazide (HCTZ).

Irbesartan is a non-peptide compound, chemically described as a 2-butyl-3-[*p*-(*o*-1*H*-tetrazol-5-ylphenyl)benzyl]-1,3-diazaspiro[4,4]non-1-en-4-one. Its empirical formula is $C_{25}H_{28}N_6O$, and its structural formula is:

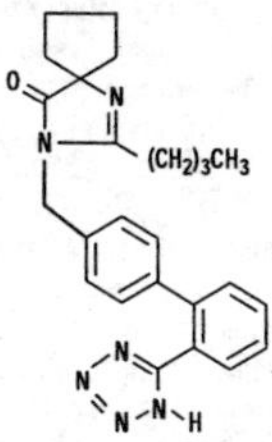

Irbesartan is a white to off-white crystalline powder with a molecular weight of 428.5. It is a nonpolar compound with a partition coefficient (octanol/water) of 10.1 at pH of 7.4. Irbesartan is slightly soluble in alcohol and methylene chloride and practically insoluble in water.

Hydrochlorothiazide is 6-chloro-3,4-dihydro- 2*H*-1,2,4-benzothiadiazine-7-sulfonamide 1,1-dioxide. Its empirical formula is $C_7H_8ClN_3O_4S_2$ and its structural formula is:

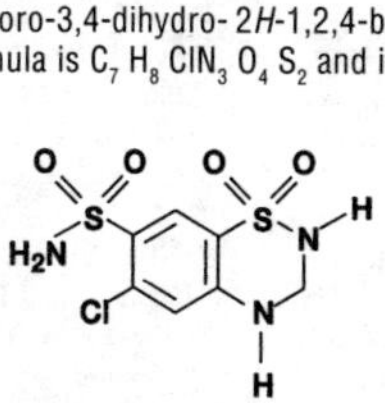

*Registered trademark of Sanofi-Synthelabo, Inc.

Hydrochlorothiazide is a white, or practically white, crystalline powder with a molecular weight of 297.7. Hydrochlorothiazide is slightly soluble in water and freely soluble in sodium hydroxide solution.

AVAPRO is available for oral administration in unscored tablets containing 75 mg, 150 mg, or 300 mg of irbesartan. Inactive ingredients include: lactose, microcrystalline cellulose, pregelatinized starch, croscarmellose sodium, poloxamer 188, silicon dioxide and magnesium stearate. AVALIDE is available for oral administration in tablets containing 150 mg or 300 mg of irbesartan combined with 12.5 mg of hydrochlorothiazide. Inactive ingredients include: lactose monohydrate, microcrystalline cellulose, pregelatinized starch, croscarmellose sodium, ferric oxide red, ferric oxide yellow, silicon dioxide, and magnesium stearate.

CLINICAL PHARMACOLOGY

Mechanism Of Action

Irbesartan

Angiotensin II is a potent vasoconstrictor formed from angiotensin I in a reaction catalyzed by angiotensin-converting enzyme (ACE, kininase II). Angiotensin II is the principal pressor agent of the renin-angiotensin system (RAS) and also stimulates aldosterone synthesis and secretion by adrenal cortex, cardiac contraction, renal resorption of sodium, activity of the sympathetic nervous system, and smooth muscle cell growth. Irbesartan blocks the vasoconstrictor and aldosterone-secreting effects of angiotensin II by selectively binding to the AT_1 angiotensin II receptor. There is also an AT_2 receptor in many tissues, but it is not involved in cardiovascular homeostasis.

Irbesartan is a specific competitive antagonist of AT_1 receptors with a much greater affinity (more than 8500-fold) for the AT_1 receptor than for the AT_2 receptor, and no agonist activity.

Blockade of the AT_1 receptor removes the negative feedback of angiotensin II on renin secretion, but the resulting increased plasma renin activity and circulating angiotensin II do not overcome the effects of irbesartan on blood pressure.

Irbesartan does not inhibit ACE or renin or affect other hormone receptors or ion channels known to be involved in the cardiovascular regulation of blood pressure and sodium homeostasis. Because irbesartan does not inhibit ACE, it does not affect the response to bradykinin; whether this has clinical relevance is not known.

Hydrochlorothiazide

Hydrochlorothiazide is a thiazide diuretic. Thiazides affect the renal tubular mechanisms of electrolyte reabsorption, directly increasing excretion of sodium and chloride in approximately equivalent amounts. Indirectly, the diuretic action of hydrochlorothiazide reduces plasma volume, with consequent increases in plasma renin activity, increases in aldosterone secretion, increases in urinary potassium loss, and decreases in serum potassium. The renin-aldosterone link is mediated by angiotensin II, so coadministration of an angiotensin II receptor antagonist tends to reverse the potassium loss associated with these diuretics.

The mechanism of the antihypertensive effect of thiazides is not fully understood.

Pharmacokinetics

Irbesartan

Irbesartan is an orally active agent that does not require biotransformation into an active form. The oral absorption of irbesartan is rapid and complete with an average absolute bioavailability of 60–80%. Following oral administration of irbesartan, peak plasma concentrations of irbesartan are attained at 1.5–2 hours after dosing. Food does not affect the bioavailability of irbesartan.

Irbesartan exhibits linear pharmacokinetics over the therapeutic dose range.

The terminal elimination half-life of irbesartan averaged 11–15 hours. Steady-state concentrations are achieved within 3 days. Limited accumulation of irbesartan (<20%) is observed in plasma upon repeated once-daily dosing.

Hydrochlorothiazide
When plasma levels have been followed for at least 24 hours, the plasma half-life has been observed to vary between 5.6 and 14.8 hours.

Metabolism and Elimination
Irbesartan
Irbesartan is metabolized via glucuronide conjugation and oxidation. Following oral or intravenous administration of ^{14}C-labeled irbesartan, more than 80% of the circulating plasma radioactivity is attributable to unchanged irbesartan. The primary circulating metabolite is the inactive irbesartan glucuronide conjugate (approximately 6%). The remaining oxidative metabolites do not add appreciably to irbesartan's pharmacologic activity.

Irbesartan and its metabolites are excreted by both biliary and renal routes. Following either oral or intravenous administration of ^{14}C-labeled irbesartan, about 20% of radioactivity is recovered in the urine and the remainder in the feces, as irbesartan or irbesartan glucuronide.

In vitro studies of irbesartan oxidation by cytochrome P450 isoenzymes indicated irbesartan was oxidized primarily by 2C9; metabolism by 3A4 was negligible. Irbesartan was neither metabolized by, nor did it substantially induce or inhibit, isoenzymes commonly associated with drug metabolism (1A1, 1A2, 2A6, 2B6, 2D6, 2E1). There was no induction or inhibition of 3A4.

Hydrochlorothiazide
Hydrochlorothiazide is not metabolized but is eliminated rapidly by the kidney. At least 61 percent of the oral dose is eliminated unchanged within 24 hours.

Distribution
Irbesartan
Irbesartan is 90% bound to serum proteins (primarily albumin and α_1-acid glycoprotein) with negligible binding to cellular components of blood. The average volume of distribution is 53–93 liters. Total plasma and renal clearances are in the range of 157–176 and 3.0–3.5 mL/min, respectively. With repetitive dosing, irbesartan accumulates to no clinically relevant extent.

Studies in animals indicate that radiolabeled irbesartan weakly crosses the blood brain barrier and placenta. Irbesartan is excreted in the milk of lactating rats.

Hydrochlorothiazide
Hydrochlorothiazide crosses the placenta but not the blood-brain barrier and is excreted in breast milk.

Special Populations
Pediatric: The pharmacokinetics of irbesartan were studied in hypertensive children (age 6–12, n=9) and adolescents (age 13–16, n=12) following single and multiple daily doses of 2 mg/kg (maximum dose of 150 mg per day) for 4 weeks. Accumulation with repeated doses was limited (18%) in both age groups. Clearance rates, AUC values, and C_{max} values were comparable to adults receiving 150 mg daily. Irbesartan pharmacokinetics have not been investigated in patients <6 years of age.

Gender: No gender related differences in pharmacokinetics were observed in healthy elderly (age 65–80 years) or in healthy young (age 18–40 years) subjects. In studies of hypertensive patients, there was no gender difference in half-life or accumulation, but somewhat higher plasma concentrations of irbesartan were observed in females (11–44%). No gender-related dosage adjustment is necessary.

Geriatric: In elderly subjects (age 65–80 years), irbesartan elimination half-life was not significantly altered, but AUC and C_{max} values were about 20–50% greater than those of young subjects (age 18–40 years). No dosage adjustment is necessary in the elderly.

Race: In healthy black subjects, irbesartan AUC values were approximately 25% greater than whites; there were no differences in C_{max} values.

Renal Insufficiency: The pharmacokinetics of irbesartan were not altered in patients with renal impairment or in patients on hemodialysis. Irbesartan is not removed by hemodialysis. No dosage adjustment is necessary in patients with mild to severe renal impairment unless a patient with renal impairment is also volume depleted. (See **WARNINGS: Hypotension in Volume- or Salt-depleted Patients** and **DOSAGE AND ADMINISTRATION**.)

Hepatic Insufficiency: The pharmacokinetics of irbesartan following repeated oral administration were not significantly affected in patients with mild to moderate cirrhosis of the liver. No dosage adjustment is necessary in patients with hepatic insufficiency.

Drug Interactions: (See **PRECAUTIONS: Drug Interactions**.)

Pharmacodynamics

Irbesartan

In healthy subjects, single oral irbesartan doses of up to 300 mg produced dose-dependent inhibition of the pressor effect of angiotensin II infusions. Inhibition was complete (100%) 4 hours following oral doses of 150 mg or 300 mg and partial inhibition was sustained for 24 hours (60% and 40% at 300 mg and 150 mg, respectively).

In hypertensive patients, angiotensin II receptor inhibition following chronic administration of irbesartan causes a 1.5–2 fold rise in angiotensin II plasma concentration and a 2–3 fold increase in plasma renin levels. Aldosterone plasma concentrations generally decline following irbesartan administration, but serum potassium levels are not significantly affected at recommended doses.

In hypertensive patients, chronic oral doses of irbesartan (up to 300 mg) had no effect on glomerular filtration rate, renal plasma flow or filtration fraction. In multiple dose studies in hypertensive patients, there were no clinically important effects on fasting triglycerides, total cholesterol, HDL-cholesterol, or fasting glucose concentrations. There was no effect on serum uric acid during chronic oral administration and no uricosuric effect.

Hydrochlorothiazide

After oral administration of hydrochlorothiazide, diuresis begins within 2 hours, peaks in about 4 hours and lasts about 6 to 12 hours.

Clinical Studies

Irbesartan

The antihypertensive effects of irbesartan were examined in seven (7) major placebo-controlled 8–12 week trials in patients with baseline diastolic blood pressures of 95–110 mmHg. Doses of 1–900 mg were included in these trials in order to fully explore the dose-range of irbesartan. These studies allowed a comparison of once- or twice-daily regimens at 150 mg/day, comparisons of peak and trough effects, and comparisons of response by gender, age, and race. Two of the seven placebo-controlled trials identified above and two additional placebo-controlled studies examined the antihypertensive effects of irbesartan and hydrochlorothiazide in combination.

The seven (7) studies of irbesartan monotherapy included a total of 1915 patients randomized to irbesartan (1–900 mg) and 611 patients randomized to placebo. Once-daily doses of 150 to 300 mg provided statistically and clinically significant decreases in systolic and diastolic blood pressure with trough (24 hour post-dose) effects after 6–12 weeks of treatment compared to placebo, of about 8–10/5–6 and 8–12/5–8 mmHg, respectively. No further increase in effect was seen at dosages greater than 300 mg. The dose-response relationships for effects on systolic and diastolic pressure are shown in Figures 1 and 2.

Once-daily administration of therapeutic doses of irbesartan gave peak effects at around 3–6 hours and, in one continuous ambulatory blood pressure monitoring study, and again around 14 hours. This was seen with both once-daily and twice-daily dosing. Trough-to-peak ratios for systolic and diastolic response were generally between 60–70%. In a continuous ambulatory blood pressure monitoring study, once-daily dosing with 150 mg gave trough and mean 24-hour responses similar to those observed in patients receiving twice-daily dosing at the same total daily dose.

In controlled trials, the addition of irbesartan to hydrochlorothiazide doses of 6.25, 12.5, or 25 mg produced further dose-related reductions in blood pressure similar to those achieved with the same monotherapy dose of irbesartan. HCTZ also had an approximately additive effect.

Analysis of age, gender, and race subgroups of patients showed that men and women, and patients over and under 65 years of age, had generally similar responses. Irbesartan was effective in reducing blood pressure regardless of race, although the effect was somewhat less in blacks (usually a low-renin population). Black patients typically show an improved response with the addition of a low dose diuretic (e.g., 12.5 mg hydrochlorothiazide).

The effect of irbesartan is apparent after the first dose and is close to the full observed effect at 2 weeks. At the end of the 8-week exposure, about 2/3 of the antihypertensive effect was still present 1 week after the last dose. Rebound hypertension was not observed. There was essentially no change in average heart rate in irbesartan-treated patients in controlled trials.

Figure 1.
Placebo-subtracted reduction in trough SeSBP; integrated analysis

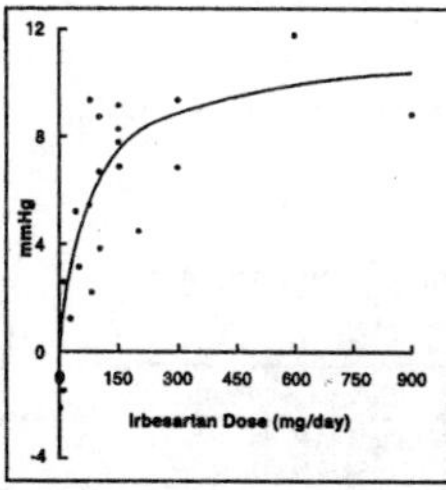

Figure 2.
Placebo-subtracted reduction in trough SeDBP; integrated analysis

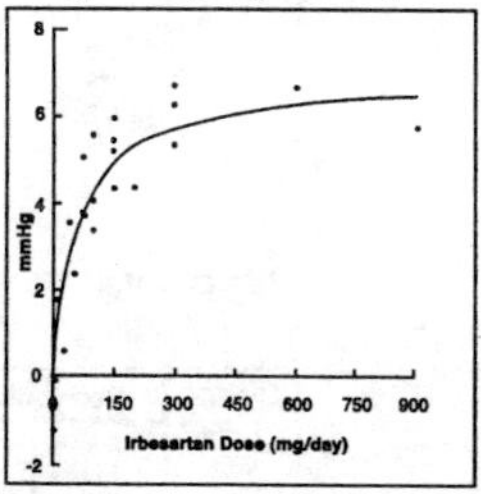

Nephropathy in Type 2 Diabetic Patients:

The Irbesartan Diabetic Nephropathy Trial (IDNT) was a randomized, placebo- and active-controlled, double-blind multicenter study, conducted worldwide in 1715 patients with type 2 diabetes, hypertension (SeSBP >135 mmHg or SeDBP >85 mmHg), and nephropathy (serum creatinine 1.0 to 3.0 mg/dL in females or 1.2 to 3.0 mg/dL in males and proteinuria ≥900 mg/day). Patients were randomized to receive AVAPRO (irbesartan) 75 mg, amlodipine 2.5 mg, or matching placebo, once-daily. Patients were titrated to a maintenance dose of AVAPRO 300 mg, or amlodipine 10 mg, as tolerated. Additional antihypertensive agents (excluding ACE inhibitors, angiotensin II receptor antagonists and calcium channel blockers) were added as needed to achieve blood pressure goal (≤135/85 or 10 mmHg reduction in systolic blood pressure if higher than 160 mmHg) for patients in all groups.

The study population was 66.5% male, 72.9% below 65 years of age and 72% White, (Asian/Pacific Islander 5.0%, Black 13.3%, Hispanic 4.8%). The mean baseline seated systolic and diastolic blood pressure were 159 mmHg and 87 mmHg, respectively. The patients entered the trial with a mean serum creatinine of 1.67 mg/dL and mean proteinuria of 4144 mg/day.

The mean blood pressure achieved was 142/77 mmHg for AVAPRO, 142/76 mmHg for amlodipine, and 145/79 mmHg for placebo. Overall, 83.0% of patients received the target dose of irbesartan more than 50% of the time. Patients were followed for a mean duration of 2.6 years.

The primary composite endpoint was the time to occurrence of any one of the following events: doubling of baseline serum creatinine, end-stage renal disease (ESRD; defined by serum creatinine ≥6 mg/dL, dialysis, or renal transplantation) or death. Treatment with AVAPRO resulted in a 20% risk reduction versus placebo (p=0.0234) (see Figure 3 and Table 1). Treatment with AVAPRO also reduced the occurrence of sustained doubling of serum creatinine as a separate end point (33%), but had no significant effect on ESRD alone and no effect on overall mortality (See Table 1).

Figure 3.
IDNT: Kaplan-Meier Estimates of Primary Endpoint
(Doubling of Serum Creatinine, End-Stage Renal Disease or All-Cause Mortality)

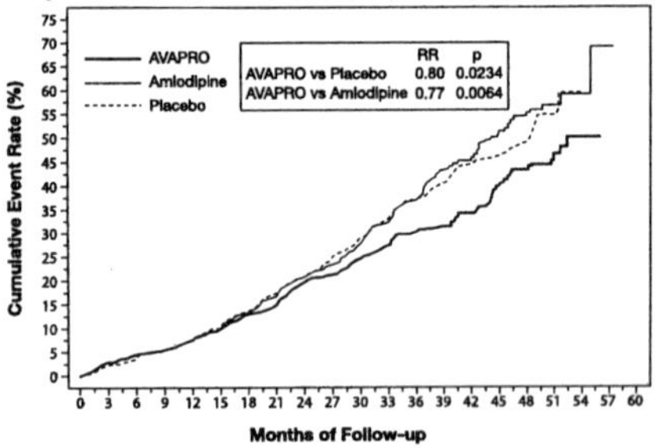

The percentages of patients experiencing an event during the course of the study can be seen in **Table 1** below.

Table 1.
IDNT: Components of Primary Composite Endpoint

	AVAPRO	Comparison with placebo			Comparison with amlodipine		
	N=579 (%)	Placebo N=569 (%)	Hazard Ratio	95% CI	Amlodipine N=567 (%)	Hazard Ratio	95% CI
Primary Composite Endpoint	32.6	39.0	0.80	0.66-0.97 (p=0.0234)	41.1	0.77	0.63-0.93
Breakdown of first occurring event contributing to primary endpoint							
2x creatinine	14.2	19.5	—	—	22.8	—	—
ESRD	7.4	8.3	—	—	8.8	—	—
Death	11.1	11.2	—	—	9.5	—	—
Incidence of total events over entire period of follow-up							
2x creatinine	16.9	23.7	0.67	0.52-0.87	25.4	0.63	0.49-0.81
ESRD	14.2	17.8	0.77	0.57-1.03	18.3	0.77	0.57-1.03
Death	15.0	16.3	0.92	0.69-1.23	14.6	1.04	0.77-1.40

The secondary endpoint of the study was a composite of cardiovascular mortality and morbidity (myocardial infarction, hospitalization for heart failure, stroke with permanent neurological deficit, amputation). There were no statistically significant differences among treatment groups in these endpoints. Compared with placebo, AVAPRO (irbesartan) significantly reduced proteinuria by about 27%, an effect that was evident within 3 months of starting therapy. AVAPRO significantly reduced the rate of loss of renal function (glomerular filtration rate), as measured by the reciprocal of the serum creatinine concentration, by 18.2%.

Table 2 presents results for demographic subgroups. Subgroup analyses are difficult to interpret and it is not known whether these observations represent true differences or chance effects. For the primary endpoint, AVAPRO's favorable effects were seen in patients also taking other antihypertensive medications (angiotensin II receptor antagonists, angiotensin converting enzyme inhibitors and calcium channel blockers were not allowed), oral hypoglycemic agents, and lipid-lowering agents.

Table 2.
IDNT: Primary Efficacy Outcome Within Subgroups

Baseline Factors	AVAPRO N=579 (%)	Comparison with placebo		
		Placebo N=569 (%)	Hazard Ratio	95% CI
Gender				
Male	27.5	36.7	0.68	0.53-0.88
Female	42.3	44.6	0.98	0.72-1.34
Race				
White	29.5	37.3	0.75	0.60-0.95
Non-White	42.6	43.5	0.95	0.67-1.34
Age (years)				
<65	31.8	39.9	0.77	0.62-0.97
≥65	35.1	36.8	0.88	0.61-1.29

Irbesartan-Hydrochlorothiazide
The antihypertensive effects of AVALIDE (irbesartan-hydrochlorothiazide) Tablets were examined in 4 placebo-controlled studies of 8–12 weeks in patients with mild-moderate hypertension. These trials included 1914 patients randomized to fixed doses of irbesartan (37.5 to 300 mg) and concomitant hydrochlorothiazide (6.25 to 25 mg). One factorial study compared all combinations of irbesartan (37.5, 100 and 300 mg or placebo) and hydrochlorothiazide (6.25, 12.5, and 25 mg or placebo). The irbesartan-hydrochlorothiazide combinations of 75/12.5 mg and 150/12.5 mg were compared to their individual components and placebo in a separate study. A third study investigated the ambulatory blood pressure responses to irbesartan-hydrochlorothiazide (75/12.5 mg and 150/12.5 mg) and placebo after 8 weeks of dosing. Another trial investigated the effects of the addition of irbesartan (75 mg) in patients not controlled on hydrochlorothiazide (25 mg) alone.

In controlled trials, the addition of irbesartan 150–300 mg to hydrochlorothiazide doses of 6.25, 12.5 or 25 mg produced further dose-related reductions in blood pressure of 8–10/3–6 mmHg, comparable to those achieved with the same monotherapy dose of irbesartan. The addition of hydrochlorothiazide to irbesartan produced further dose-related reductions in blood pressure at trough (24 hours post-dose) of 5–6/2–3 mmHg (12.5 mg) and 7–11/4–5 mmHg (25 mg), also comparable to effects achieved with hydrochlorothiazide alone. Once-daily dosing with 150 mg irbesartan and 12.5 mg hydrochlorothiazide, 300 mg irbesartan and 12.5 mg hydrochlorothiazide, or 300 mg irbesartan and 25 mg hydrochlorothiazide produced mean placebo-adjusted blood pressure reductions at trough (24 hours post-dosing) of about 13–15/7–9, 14/9–12, and 19–21/11–12 mmHg, respectively. Peak effects occurred at 3–6 hours, with the trough-to-peak ratios >65%.

In another study, irbesartan (75–150 mg) or placebo was added on a background of 25 mg hydrochlorothiazide in patients not adequately controlled (SeDBP 93–120 mmHg) on hydrochlorothiazide (25 mg) alone. The addition of irbesartan (75–150 mg) gave an additive effect (systolic/diastolic) at trough (24 hours post-dosing) of 11/7 mmHg.

There was no difference in response for men and women or in patients over or under 65 years of age. Black patients had a larger response to hydrochlorothiazide than non-black patients and a smaller response to irbesartan. The overall response to the combination was similar for black and non-black patients.

INDICATIONS AND USAGE
Hypertension
AVAPRO (irbesartan) is indicated for the treatment of hypertension. It may be used alone or in combination with other antihypertensive agents. AVALIDE (irbesartan-hydrochlorothiazide) Tablets is indicated for the treatment of hypertension. This fixed dose combination is not indicated for initial therapy (see **DOSAGE AND ADMINISTRATION**).

Nephropathy in Type 2 Diabetic Patients
AVAPRO is indicated for the treatment of diabetic nephropathy with an elevated serum creatinine and proteinuria (>300 mg/day) in patients with type 2 diabetes and hypertension. In this population, AVAPRO reduces the rate of progression of nephropathy as measured by the occurrence of doubling serum creatinine or end stage renal disease (need for dialysis or renal transplantation) (See **CLINICAL PHARMACOLOGY: Clinical Studies**).

CONTRAINDICATIONS
AVAPRO and AVALIDE are contraindicated in patients who are hypersensitive to any component of these products.

Because of the hydrochlorothiazide component, AVALIDE is contraindicated in patients with anuria or hypersensitivity to other sulfonamide-derived drugs.

WARNINGS
Fetal/Neonatal Morbidity and Mortality
Drugs that act directly on the renin-angiotensin system can cause fetal and neonatal morbidity and death when administered to pregnant women. Several dozen cases have been reported in the world literature in patients who were taking angiotensin converting enzyme inhibitors. When pregnancy is detected, AVAPRO and AVALIDE Tablets should be discontinued as soon as possible.

The use of drugs that act directly on the renin-angiotensin system during the second and third trimesters of pregnancy has been associated with fetal and neonatal injury, including hypotension, neonatal skull hypoplasia, anuria, reversible or irreversible renal failure, and death. Oligohydramnios has also been reported, presumably resulting from decreased fetal renal function; oligohydramnios in this setting has been associated with fetal limb contractures, craniofacial deformation, and hypoplastic lung development. Prematurity, intrauterine growth retardation, and patent ductus arteriosus have also been reported, although it is not clear whether these occurrences were due to exposure to the drug.

These adverse effects do not appear to have resulted from intrauterine drug exposure that has been limited to the first trimester.

Mothers whose embryos and fetuses are exposed to an angiotensin II receptor antagonist only during the first trimester should be so informed. Nonetheless, when patients become pregnant, physicians should have the patient discontinue the use of AVAPRO (irbesartan) and AVALIDE (irbesartan-hydrochlorothiazide)as soon as possible.

Rarely (probably less often than once in every thousand pregnancies), no alternative to a drug acting on the renin-angiotensin system will be found. In these rare cases, the mothers should be apprised of the potential hazards to their fetuses, and serial ultrasound examinations should be performed to assess the intraamniotic environment.

If oligohydramnios is observed, AVAPRO and AVALIDE should be discontinued unless it is considered life-saving for the mother. Contraction stress testing (CST), a non-stress test (NST), or biophysical profiling (BPP) may be appropriate depending upon the week of pregnancy. Patients and physicians should be aware, however, that oligohydramnios may not appear until after the fetus has sustained irreversible injury.

Infants with histories of *in utero* exposure to an angiotensin II receptor antagonist should be closely observed for hypotension, oliguria, and hyperkalemia. If oliguria occurs, attention should be directed toward support of blood pressure and renal perfusion. Exchange transfusion or dialysis may be required as a means of reversing hypotension and/or substituting for disordered renal function.

When pregnant rats were treated with irbesartan from day 0 to day 20 of gestation (oral doses of 50, 180, and 650 mg/kg/day), increased incidences of renal pelvic cavitation, hydroureter and/or absence of renal papilla were observed in fetuses at doses ≥50 mg/kg/day [approximately equivalent to the maximum recommended human dose (MRHD), 300 mg/day, on a body surface area basis]. Subcutaneous edema was observed in fetuses at doses ≥180 mg/kg/day (about 4 times the MRHD on a body surface area basis). As these anomalies were not observed in rats in which irbesartan exposure (oral doses of 50, 150 and 450 mg/kg/day) was limited to gestation days 6–15, they appear to reflect late gestational effects of the drug. In pregnant rabbits, oral doses of 30 mg irbesartan/kg/day were associated with maternal mortality and abortion. Surviving females receiving this dose (about 1.5 times the MRHD on a body surface area basis) had a slight increase in early resorptions and a corresponding decrease in live fetuses. Irbesartan was found to cross the placental barrier in rats and rabbits.

Radioactivity was present in the rat and rabbit fetus during late gestation and in rat milk following oral doses of radiolabeled irbesartan.

Studies in which hydrochlorothiazide was administered to pregnant mice and rats during their respective periods of major organogenesis at doses up to 3000 and 1000 mg/kg/day, respectively, provided no evidence of harm to the fetus.

A development toxicity study was performed in rats with doses of 50/50 and 150/150 mg/kg/day irbesartan-hydrochlorothiazide. Although the high dose combination appeared to be more toxic to the dams than either drug alone, there did not appear to be an increase in toxicity to the developing embryos.

Thiazides cross the placental barrier and appear in cord blood. There is a risk of fetal or neonatal jaundice, thrombocytopenia, and possibly other adverse reactions that have occurred in adults.

Hypotension in Volume- or Salt-depleted Patients

Excessive reduction of blood pressure was rarely seen in patients with uncomplicated hypertension treated with irbesartan alone (<0.1%) or with irbesartan-hydrochlorothiazide (approximately 1%). Initiation of antihypertensive therapy may cause symptomatic hypotension in patients with intravascular volume- or sodium-depletion, e.g., in patients treated vigorously with diuretics or in patients on dialysis. Such volume depletion should be corrected prior to administration of antihypertensive therapy, or a low starting dose of AVAPRO (irbesartan) should be used (see **DOSAGE AND ADMINISTRATION**).

If hypotension occurs, the patient should be placed in the supine position and, if necessary, given an intravenous infusion of normal saline. A transient hypotensive response is not a contraindication to further treatment, which usually can be continued without difficulty once the blood pressure has stabilized.

Hydrochlorothiazide

Hepatic Impairment

Thiazides should be used with caution in patients with impaired hepatic function or progressive liver disease, since minor alterations of fluid and electrolyte balance may precipitate hepatic coma.

Hypersensitivity Reaction

Hypersensitivity reactions to hydrochlorothiazide may occur in patients with or without a history of allergy or bronchial asthma, but are more likely in patients with such a history.

Systemic Lupus Erythematosus

Thiazide diuretics have been reported to cause exacerbation or activation of systemic lupus erythematosus.

Lithium Interaction

Lithium generally should not be given with thiazides (see **PRECAUTIONS: Drug Interactions**; *Hydrochlorothiazide, Lithium*).

PRECAUTIONS

General

Irbesartan-Hydrochlorothiazide

In double-blind clinical trials of various doses of irbesartan and hydrochlorothiazide, the incidence of hypertensive patients who developed hypokalemia (serum potassium <3.5 mEq/L) was 7.5% versus 6.0% for placebo; the incidence of hyperkalemia (serum potassium >5.7 mEq/L) was <1.0% versus 1.7% for placebo. No patient discontinued due to increases or decreases in serum potassium. Overall, the combination of irbesartan and hydrochlorothiazide had no effect on serum potassium. Higher doses of irbesartan ameliorated the hypokalemic response to hydrochlorothiazide.

Hydrochlorothiazide

Periodic determination of serum electrolytes to detect possible electrolyte imbalance should be performed at appropriate intervals. All patients receiving thiazide therapy should be observed for clinical signs of fluid or electrolyte imbalance: hyponatremia, hypochloremic alkalosis, and hypokalemia. Serum and urine electrolyte determinations are particularly important when the patient is vomiting excessively or receiving parenteral fluids. Warning signs or symptoms of fluid and electrolyte imbalance, irrespective of cause, include dryness of mouth, thirst, weakness, lethargy, drowsiness, restlessness, confusion, seizures, muscle pains or cramps, muscular fatigue, hypotension, oliguria, tachycardia, and gastrointestinal disturbances such as nausea and vomiting.

Hypokalemia may develop, especially with brisk diuresis, when severe cirrhosis is present, or after prolonged therapy.

Interference with adequate oral electrolyte intake will also contribute to hypokalemia. Hypokalemia may cause cardiac arrhythmia and may also sensitize or exaggerate the response of the heart to the toxic effects of digitalis (e.g., increased ventricular irritability).

Although any chloride deficit is generally mild and usually does not require specific treatment except under extraordinary circumstances (as in liver disease or renal disease), chloride replacement may be required in the treatment of metabolic alkalosis.

Dilutional hyponatremia may occur in edematous patients in hot weather; appropriate therapy is water restriction, rather than administration of salt except in rare instances when the hyponatremia is life-threatening. In actual salt depletion, appropriate replacement is the therapy of choice.

Hyperuricemia may occur or frank gout may be precipitated in certain patients receiving thiazide therapy.

In diabetic patients dosage adjustments of insulin or oral hypoglycemic agents may be required. Hyperglycemia may occur with thiazide diuretics. Thus latent diabetes mellitus may become manifest during thiazide therapy.

The antihypertensive effects of the drug may be enhanced in the post sympathectomy patient.

If progressive renal impairment becomes evident consider withholding or discontinuing diuretic therapy.

Thiazides have been shown to increase the urinary excretion of magnesium; this may result in hypomagnesemia.

Thiazides may decrease urinary calcium excretion. Thiazides may cause intermittent and slight elevation of serum calcium in the absence of known disorders of calcium metabolism. Marked hypercalcemia may be evidence of hidden hyperparathyroidism. Thiazides should be discontinued before carrying out tests for parathyroid function.

Increases in cholesterol and triglyceride levels may be associated with thiazide diuretic therapy.

Impaired Renal Function

As a consequence of inhibiting the renin-angiotensin-aldosterone system, changes in renal function may be anticipated in susceptible individuals. In patients whose renal function may depend on the activity of the renin-angiotensin-aldosterone system (e.g., patients with severe congestive heart failure), treatment with angiotensin converting enzyme inhibitors has been associated with oliguria and/or progressive azotemia and (rarely) with acute renal failure and/or death. Irbesartan would be expected to behave similarly.

In studies of ACE inhibitors in patients with unilateral or bilateral renal artery stenosis, increases in serum creatinine or BUN have been reported. There has been no known use of irbesartan in patients with unilateral or bilateral renal artery stenosis, but a similar effect should be anticipated.

Thiazides should be used with caution in severe renal disease. In patients with renal disease, thiazides may precipitate azotemia. Cumulative effects of the drug may develop in patients with impaired renal function.

Information For Patients

Pregnancy: Female patients of childbearing age should be told about the consequences of second- and third-trimester exposure to drugs that act on the renin-angiotensin system, and they should also be told that these consequences do not appear to have resulted from intrauterine drug exposure that has been limited to the first trimester. These patients should be asked to report pregnancies to their physicians as soon as possible.

Symptomatic Hypotension: A patient receiving AVALIDE (irbesartan-hydrochlorothiazide) Tablets should be cautioned that lightheadedness can occur, especially during the first days of therapy, and that it should be reported to the prescribing physician. The patients should be told that if syncope occurs, AVALIDE should be discontinued until the physician has been consulted.

All patients should be cautioned that inadequate fluid intake, excessive perspiration, diarrhea, or vomiting can lead to an excessive fall in blood pressure, with the same consequences of lightheadedness and possible syncope.

Drug Interactions

Irbesartan

No significant drug-drug pharmacokinetic (or pharmacodynamic) interactions have been found in interaction studies with hydrochlorothiazide, digoxin, warfarin, and nifedipine.

In vitro studies show significant inhibition of the formation of oxidized irbesartan metabolites with the known cytochrome CYP 2C9 substrates/inhibitors sulphenazole, tolbutamide and nifedipine. However, in clinical studies the consequences of concomitant irbesartan on the pharmacodynamics of warfarin were negligible. Concomitant nifedipine or hydrochlorothiazide had no effect on irbesartan pharmacokinetics. Based on *in vitro* data, no interaction would be expected with drugs whose metabolism is dependent upon cytochrome P450 isozymes 1A1, 1A2, 2A6, 2B6, 2D6, 2E1, or 3A4.

In separate studies of patients receiving maintenance doses of warfarin, hydrochlorothiazide, or digoxin, irbesartan administration for 7 days had no effect on the pharmacodynamics of warfarin (prothrombin time) or the pharmacokinetics of digoxin. The pharmacokinetics of irbesartan were not affected by coadministration of nifedipine or hydrochlorothiazide.

Hydrochlorothiazide

When administered concurrently the following drugs may interact with thiazide diuretics:

Alcohol, Barbiturates, Or Narcotics — potentiation of orthostatic hypotension may occur.

Antidiabetic Drugs (oral agents and insulin) — dosage adjustment of the antidiabetic drug may be required.

Other Antihypertensive Drugs — additive effect or potentiation.

Cholestyramine And Colestipol Resins — absorption of hydrochlorothiazide is impaired in the presence of anionic exchange resins. Single doses of either cholestyramine or colestipol resins bind the hydrochlorothiazide and reduce its absorption from the gastrointestinal tract by up to 85 and 43 percent, respectively.

Corticosteroids, ACTH — intensified electrolyte depletion, particularly hypokalemia.

Pressor Amines (*e.g., Norepinephrine*) — possible decreased response to pressor amines but not sufficient to preclude their use.

Skeletal Muscle Relaxants, Nondepolarizing (e.g., Tubocurarine) — possible increased responsiveness to the muscle relaxant.

Lithium — should not generally be given with diuretics. Diuretic agents reduce the renal clearance of lithium and add a high risk of lithium toxicity. Refer to the package insert for lithium preparations before use of such preparations with AVALIDE (irbesartan-hydrochlorothiazide).

Non-steroidal Anti-inflammatory Drugs — in some patients, the administration of a non-steroidal anti-inflammatory agent can reduce the diuretic, natriuretic, and antihypertensive effects of loop, potassium-sparing and thiazide diuretics. Therefore, when AVALIDE Tablets and non-steroidal anti-inflammatory agents are used concomitantly, the patient should be observed closely to determine if the desired effect of the diuretic is obtained.

Carcinogenesis, Mutagenesis, Impairment Of Fertility
Irbesartan
No evidence of carcinogenicity was observed when irbesartan was administered at doses of up to 500/1000 mg/kg/day (males/females, respectively) in rats and 1000 mg/kg/day in mice for up to two years. For male and female rats, 500 mg/kg/day provided an average systemic exposure to irbesartan ($AUC_{0-24hours}$, bound plus unbound) about 3 and 11 times, respectively, the average systemic exposure in humans receiving the maximum recommended dose (MRD) of 300 mg irbesartan/day, whereas 1000 mg/kg/day (administered to females only) provided an average systemic exposure about 21 times that reported for humans at the MRD. For male and female mice, 1000 mg/kg/day provided an exposure to irbesartan about 3 and 5 times, respectively, the human exposure at 300 mg/day.

Irbesartan was not mutagenic in a battery of *in vitro* tests (Ames microbial test, rat hepatocyte DNA repair test, V79 mammalian-cell forward gene-mutation assay). Irbesartan was negative in several tests for induction of chromosomal aberrations (*in vitro*-human lymphocyte assay; *in vivo*-mouse micronucleus study).

Irbesartan had no adverse effects on fertility or mating of male or female rats at oral doses ≤650 mg/kg/day, the highest dose providing a systemic exposure to irbesartan ($AUC_{0-24hours}$, bound plus unbound) about 5 times that found in humans receiving the maximum recommended dose of 300 mg/day.

Irbesartan-Hydrochlorothiazide
No carcinogenicity studies have been conducted with the irbesartan-hydrochlorothiazide combination.

Irbesartan-hydrochlorothiazide was not mutagenic in standard *in vitro* tests (Ames microbial test and Chinese hamster mammalian-cell forward gene-mutation assay). Irbesartan-hydrochlorothiazide was negative in tests for induction of chromosomal aberrations (*in vitro* — human lymphocyte assay; *in vivo* — mouse micronucleus study).

The combination of irbesartan and hydrochlorothiazide has not been evaluated in definitive studies of fertility.

Hydrochlorothiazide
Two-year feeding studies in mice and rats conducted under the auspices of the National Toxicology Program (NTP) uncovered no evidence of a carcinogenic potential of hydrochlorothiazide in female mice (at doses of up to approximately 600 mg/kg/day) or in male and female rats (at doses of up to approximately 100 mg/kg/day). The NTP, however, found equivocal evidence for hepatocarcinogenicity in male mice.

Hydrochlorothiazide was not genotoxic *in vitro* in the Ames mutagenicity assay of *Salmonella typhimurium* strains TA 98, TA 100, TA 1535, TA 1537, and TA 1538 and in the Chinese Hamster Ovary (CHO) test for chromosomal aberrations, or *in vivo* in assays using mouse germinal cell chromosomes, Chinese hamster bone marrow chromosomes, and the *Drosophila* sex-linked recessive lethal trait gene. Positive test results were obtained only in the *in vitro* CHO Sister Chromatid Exchange (clastogenicity) and in the Mouse Lymphoma Cell (mutagenicity) assays, using concentrations of hydrochlorothiazide from 43 to 1300 µg/mL, and in the *Aspergillus nidulans* non-disjunction assay at an unspecified concentration.

Hydrochlorothiazide had no adverse effects on the fertility of mice and rats of either sex in studies wherein these species were exposed, via their diet, to doses of up to 100 and 4 mg/kg, respectively, prior to mating and throughout gestation.

Pregnancy
Pregnancy Categories C (first trimester) and D (second and third trimesters)
(See **WARNINGS: Fetal/Neonatal Morbidity and Mortality**.)

Nursing Mothers
It is not known whether irbesartan is excreted in human milk, but irbesartan or some metabolite of irbesartan is secreted at low concentration in the milk of lactating rats.

Because of the potential for adverse effects on the nursing infant, a decision should be made whether to discontinue nursing or discontinue the drug, taking into account the importance of the drug to the mother.

Thiazides appear in human milk. Because of the potential for adverse effects on the nursing infant, a decision should be made whether to discontinue nursing or discontinue the drug, taking into account the importance of the drug to the mother.

Pediatric Use

Safety and effectiveness in pediatric patients have not been established.

Pharmacokinetic parameters in pediatric subjects (age 6–16, n=21) were comparable to adults. At doses up to 150 mg daily for 4 weeks, AVAPRO (irbesartan) was well tolerated in hypertensive children and adolescents (see **CLINICAL PHARMACOLOGY: Special Populations**). Blood pressure reductions were comparable to adults receiving 150 mg daily; however, greater sensitivity in some patients cannot be ruled out (see **DOSAGE AND ADMINISTRATION: Pediatric Patients**). AVAPRO has not been studied in pediatric patients less than 6 years old.

Geriatric Use

Irbesartan

Of 4925 subjects receiving AVAPRO (irbesartan) in controlled clinical studies of hypertension, 911 (18.5%) were 65 years and over, while 150 (3.0%) were 75 years and over. No overall differences in effectiveness or safety were observed between these subjects and younger subjects, but greater sensitivity of some older individuals cannot be ruled out. (See **Pharmacokinetics**, **Special Populations**, and **Clinical Studies**.)

Irbesartan-Hydrochlorothiazide

Clinical studies of AVALIDE (irbesartan-hydrochlorothiazide) did not include sufficient numbers of subjects aged 65 and over to determine whether they respond differently from younger subjects. Other reported clinical experience has not identified differences in responses between the elderly and younger patients. In general, dose selection for an elderly patient should be cautious, usually starting at the low end of the dosing range, reflecting the greater frequency of decreased hepatic, renal, or cardiac function, and of concomitant disease or other drug therapy.

ADVERSE REACTIONS

Irbesartan

Hypertension

AVAPRO has been evaluated for safety in more than 4300 patients with hypertension and about 5000 subjects overall. This experience includes 1303 patients treated for over 6 months and 407 patients for 1 year or more. Treatment with AVAPRO was well-tolerated, with an incidence of adverse events similar to placebo. These events generally were mild and transient with no relationship to the dose of AVAPRO.

In placebo-controlled clinical trials, discontinuation of therapy due to a clinical adverse event was required in 3.3 percent of patients treated with AVAPRO, versus 4.5 percent of patients given placebo.

In placebo-controlled clinical trials, the following adverse event experiences reported in at least 1% of patients treated with AVAPRO (n=1965) and at a higher incidence versus placebo (n=641), excluding those too general to be informative and those not reasonably associated with the use of drug because they were associated with the condition being treated or are very common in the treated population include: diarrhea (3% vs. 2%), dyspepsia/heartburn (2% vs. 1%), and fatigue (4% vs. 3%).

The following adverse events occurred at an incidence of 1% or greater in patients treated with irbesartan, but were at least as frequent or more frequent in patients receiving placebo: abdominal pain, anxiety/nervousness, chest pain, dizziness, edema, headache, influenza, musculoskeletal pain, pharyngitis, nausea/ vomiting, rash, rhinitis, sinus abnormality, tachycardia and urinary tract infection.

Irbesartan use was not associated with an increased incidence of dry cough, as is typically associated with ACE inhibitor use. In placebo controlled studies, the incidence of cough in irbesartan treated patients was 2.8% versus 2.7% in patients receiving placebo.

The incidence of hypotension or orthostatic hypotension was low in irbesartan treated patients (0.4%), unrelated to dosage, and similar to the incidence among placebo treated patients (0.2%). Dizziness, syncope, and vertigo were reported with equal or less frequency in patients receiving irbesartan compared with placebo.

In addition, the following potentially important events occurred in less than 1% of the 1965 patients and at least 5 patients (0.3%) receiving irbesartan in clinical studies, and those less frequent, clinically significant events (listed by body system). It cannot be determined whether these events were causally related to irbesartan:

Body as a Whole: fever, chills, facial edema, upper extremity edema;

Cardiovascular: flushing, hypertension, cardiac murmur, myocardial infarction, angina pectoris, arrhythmic/conduction disorder, cardio-respiratory arrest, heart failure, hypertensive crisis;

Dermatologic: pruritus, dermatitis, ecchymosis, erythema face, urticaria;

Endocrine/Metabolic/Electrolyte Imbalances: sexual dysfunction, libido change, gout;

Gastrointestinal: constipation, oral lesion, gastroenteritis, flatulence, abdominal distention;

Musculoskeletal/Connective Tissue: extremity swelling, muscle cramp, arthritis, muscle ache, musculoskeletal chest pain, joint stiffness, bursitis, muscle weakness;

Nervous System: sleep disturbance, numbness, somnolence, emotional disturbance, depression, paresthesia, tremor, transient ischemic attack, cerebrovascular accident;

Renal/Genitourinary: abnormal urination, prostate disorder;

Respiratory: epistaxis, tracheobronchitis, congestion, pulmonary congestion, dyspnea, wheezing;

Special Senses: vision disturbance, hearing abnormality, ear infection, ear pain, conjunctivitis, other eye disturbance, eyelid abnormality, ear abnormality.

Nephropathy in Type 2 Diabetic Patients

In clinical studies in patients with hypertension and type 2 diabetic renal disease, the adverse drug experiences were similar to those seen in patients with hypertension with the exception of an increased incidence of orthostatic symptoms (dizziness, orthostatic dizziness, and orthostatic hypotension) observed in IDNT (proteinuria ≥900 mg/day, and serum creatinine ranging from 1.0-3.0 mg/dL). In this trial, orthostatic symptoms occurred more frequently in the AVAPRO (irbesartan) group (dizziness 10.2%, orthostatic dizziness 5.4%, orthostatic hypotension 5.4%) than in the placebo group (dizziness 6.0%, orthostatic dizziness 2.7%, orthostatic hypotension 3.2%).

Irbesartan-Hydrochlorothiazide

Hypertension

AVALIDE (irbesartan-hydrochlorothiazide) Tablets have been evaluated for safety in 898 patients treated for essential hypertension. In clinical trials with AVALIDE, no adverse experiences peculiar to this combination drug product have been observed. Adverse experiences have been limited to those that were reported previously with irbesartan and/or hydrochlorothiazide (HCTZ). The overall incidence of adverse experiences reported with the combination was comparable to placebo. In general, treatment with AVALIDE was well tolerated. For the most part, adverse experiences have been mild and transient in nature and have not required discontinuation of therapy. In controlled clinical trials, discontinuation of AVALIDE therapy due to clinical adverse experiences was required in only 3.6%. This incidence was significantly less ($p=0.023$) than the 6.8% of patients treated with placebo who discontinued therapy.

In these double-blind controlled clinical trials, the following adverse experiences reported with AVALIDE occurred in ≥1% of patients, and more often on the irbesartan-hydrochlorothiazide combination than on placebo, regardless of drug relationship:

	Irbesartan/HCTZ (n=898) (%)	Placebo (n=236) (%)	Irbesartan (n=400) (%)	HCTZ (n=380) (%)
Body as a Whole				
Chest Pain	2	1	2	2
Fatigue	7	3	4	3
Influenza	3	1	2	2
Cardiovascular				
Edema	3	3	2	2
Tachycardia	1	0	1	1
Gastrointestinal				
Abdominal Pain	2	1	2	2
Dyspepsia/heartburn	2	1	0	2
Nausea/vomiting	3	0	2	0
Immunology				
Allergy	1	0	1	1
Musculoskeletal				
Musculoskeletal Pain	7	5	6	10
Nervous System				
Dizziness	8	4	6	5
Dizziness Orthostatic	1	0	1	1
Renal/Genitourinary				
Abnormality Urination	2	1	1	2

The following adverse events were also reported at a rate of 1% or greater, but were as, or more, common in the placebo group: headache, sinus abnormality, cough, URI, pharyngitis, diarrhea, rhinitis, urinary tract infection, rash, anxiety/nervousness, and muscle cramp.

Adverse events occurred at about the same rates in men and women, older and younger patients, and black and non-black patients.

Hydrochlorothiazide

Other adverse experiences that have been reported with hydrochlorothiazide, without regard to causality, are listed below:

Body As A Whole: weakness

Digestive: pancreatitis, jaundice (intrahepatic cholestatic jaundice), sialadenitis, cramping, gastric irritation

Hematologic: aplastic anemia, agranulocytosis, leukopenia, hemolytic anemia, thrombocytopenia

Hypersensitivity: purpura, photosensitivity, urticaria, necrotizing angiitis (vasculitis and cutaneous vasculitis), fever, respiratory distress including pneumonitis and pulmonary edema, anaphylactic reactions

Metabolic: hyperglycemia, glycosuria, hyperuricemia

Musculoskeletal: muscle spasm

Nervous System/Psychiatric: restlessness

Renal: renal failure, renal dysfunction, interstitial nephritis

Skin: erythema multiforme including Stevens-Johnson syndrome, exfoliative dermatitis including toxic epidermal necrolysis

Special Senses: transient blurred vision, xanthopsia.

Post-Marketing Experience

The following have been very rarely reported in post-marketing experience: urticaria, angioedema (involving swelling of the face, lips, pharynx, and/or tongue); increased liver function tests; jaundice. Hyperkalemia has been rarely reported.

Laboratory Test Findings
Hypertension
In controlled clinical trials, clinically important changes in standard laboratory parameters were rarely associated with administration of AVAPRO (irbesartan) and AVALIDE (irbesartan-hydrochlorothiazide) Tablets.

Irbesartan
Creatinine, Blood Urea Nitrogen: Minor increases in blood urea nitrogen (BUN) or serum creatinine were observed in less than 0.7% of patients with essential hypertension treated with AVAPRO alone versus 0.9% on placebo. (See **PRECAUTIONS: Impaired Renal Function**.)

Hematologic: Mean decreases in hemoglobin of 0.2 g/dL were observed in 0.2% of patients receiving AVAPRO compared to 0.3% of placebo treated patients. Neutropenia (<1000 cells/mm^3) occurred at similar frequencies among patients receiving AVAPRO (0.3%) and placebo treated patients (0.5%).

Nephropathy in Type 2 Diabetic Patients
Hyperkalemia: In IDNT (proteinuria ≥900 mg/day, and serum creatinine ranging from 1.0–3.0 mg/dL), the percent of patients with hyperkalemia (>6 mEq/L) was 18.6% in the AVAPRO group vs. 6.0% in the placebo group. Discontinuations due to hyperkalemia in the AVAPRO group were 2.1% vs. 0.4% in the placebo group.

Irbesartan-Hydrochlorothiazide
Hypertension
Creatinine, Blood Urea Nitrogen: Minor increases in blood urea nitrogen (BUN) or serum creatinine were observed in 2.3 and 1.1 %, respectively, of patients with essential hypertension treated with AVALIDE alone. No patient discontinued taking AVALIDE due to increased BUN. One patient discontinued taking AVALIDE due to a minor increase in serum creatinine.

Hemoglobin: Mean decreases of approximately 0.2 g/dL occurred in patients treated with AVALIDE alone, but were rarely of clinical importance. This compared to a mean of 0.4 g/dL in patients receiving placebo. No patients were discontinued due to anemia.

Liver Function Tests: Occasional elevations of liver enzymes and/or serum bilirubin have occurred. In patients with essential hypertension treated with AVALIDE (irbesartan-hydrochlorothiazide) alone, one patient was discontinued due to elevated liver enzymes.

Serum Electrolytes: (See **PRECAUTIONS**.)

OVERDOSAGE

Irbesartan
No data are available in regard to overdosage in humans. However, daily doses of 900 mg for 8 weeks were well-tolerated. The most likely manifestations of overdosage are expected to be hypotension and tachycardia; bradycardia might also occur from overdose. Irbesartan is not removed by hemodialysis.

To obtain up-to-date information about the treatment of overdosage, a good resource is a certified Regional Poison-Control Center. Telephone numbers of certified poison-control centers are listed in the *Physicians' Desk Reference* (PDR). In managing overdose, consider the possibilities of multiple-drug interactions, drug-drug interactions, and unusual drug kinetics in the patient.

Laboratory determinations of serum levels of irbesartan are not widely available, and such determinations have, in any event, no established role in the management of irbesartan overdose.

Acute oral toxicity studies with irbesartan in mice and rats indicated acute lethal doses were in excess of 2000 mg/kg, about 25- and 50-fold the maximum recommended human dose (300 mg) on a mg/m^2 basis, respectively.

Hydrochlorothiazide
The most common signs and symptoms of overdose observed in humans are those caused by electrolyte depletion (hypokalemia, hypochloremia, hyponatremia) and dehydration resulting from excessive diuresis. If digitalis has also been administered, hypokalemia

may accentuate cardiac arrhythmias. The degree to which hydrochlorothiazide is removed by hemodialysis has not been established. The oral LD_{50} of hydrochlorothiazide is greater than 10 g/kg in both mice and rats.

DOSAGE AND ADMINISTRATION

AVAPRO (irbesartan) and AVALIDE (irbesartan-hydrochlorothiazide) may be administered with other anithypertensive agents and with or without food.

Irbesartan

Hypertension

The recommended initial dose of AVAPRO is 150 mg once daily. Patients requiring further reduction in blood pressure should be titrated to 300 mg once daily.

A low dose of a diuretic may be added, if blood pressure is not controlled by AVAPRO alone. Hydrochlorothiazide has been shown to have an additive effect (see **CLINICAL PHARMACOLOGY: Clinical Studies**). Patients not adequately treated by the maximum dose of 300 mg once daily are unlikely to derive additional benefit from a higher dose or twice-daily dosing.

No dosage adjustment is necessary in elderly patients, or in patients with hepatic impairment or mild to severe renal impairment.

Nephropathy in Type 2 Diabetic Patients

The recommended target maintenance dose is 300 mg once daily. There are no data on the clinical effects of lower doses of AVAPRO on diabetic nephropathy (see **CLINICAL PHARMACOLOGY: Clinical Studies**).

Pediatric Patients

Children (<6 years): Safety and effectiveness have not been established.

Children (6–12 years): An initial dose of 75 mg once daily is reasonable. Patients requiring further reduction in blood pressure should be titrated to 150 mg once daily (see **PRECAUTIONS: Pediatric Use**).

Adolescent patients (13-16 years): An initial dose of 150 mg once daily is reasonable. Patients requiring further reduction in blood pressure should be titrated to 300 mg once daily. Higher doses are not recommended (see **PRECAUTIONS: Pediatric Use**).

Volume- and Salt-depleted Patients

A lower initial dose of AVAPRO (75 mg) is recommended in patients with depletion of intravascular volume or salt (e.g., patients treated vigorously with diuretics or on hemodialysis) (see **WARNINGS: Hypotension in Volume- or Salt-depleted Patients)**.

Irbesartan-Hydrochlorothiazide

Hypertension

The recommended initial dose of irbesartan is 150 mg once daily. Patients requiring further reduction in blood pressure should be titrated to 300 mg once daily.

A lower initial dose of irbesartan (75 mg) is recommended in patients with depletion of intravascular volume (e.g., patients treated vigorously with diuretics or on hemodialysis) (see **WARNING: Hypotension in Volume- or Salt-depleted Patients**). Patients not adequately treated by the maximum dose of 300 mg once daily are unlikely to derive additional benefit from a higher dose or twice-daily dosing.

Hydrochlorothiazide is effective in doses of 12.5 to 50 mg once daily.

To minimize dose-independent side effects, it is usually appropriate to begin combination therapy only after a patient has failed to achieve the desired effect with monotherapy.

The side effects (see **WARNINGS**) of irbesartan are generally rare and apparently independent of dose; those of hydrochlorothiazide are a mixture of dose-dependent (primarily hypokalemia) and dose-independent phenomena (e.g., pancreatitis), the former much more common than the latter. Therapy with any combination of irbesartan and hydrochlorothiazide will be associated with both sets of dose-independent side effects.

Replacement Therapy

The combination may be substituted for the titrated components.

Dose Titration by Clinical Effect

A patient whose blood pressure is inadequately controlled by irbesartan or hydrochlorothiazide alone may be switched to once daily AVALIDE. Recommended doses of AVALIDE, in order of increasing mean effect, are (irbesartan-hydrochlorothiazide) 150/12.5 mg, 300/12.5 mg, and 300/25 mg (two 150/12.5 mg tablets). The largest incremental effect will likely be in the transition from monotherapy to 150/12.5 mg. (See **CLINICAL PHARMACOLOGY: Clinical Studies**). It takes 2-4 weeks for the blood pressure to stabilize after a change in the dose of AVALIDE.

The usual dose of AVALIDE is one tablet once daily. More than two tablets once daily is not recommended. The maximal antihypertensive effect is attained about 2–4 weeks after initiation of therapy.

Use in Patients with Renal Impairment

The usual regimens of therapy with AVALIDE may be followed as long as the patient's creatinine clearance is >30 mL/min. In patients with more severe renal impairment, loop diuretics are preferred to thiazides, so AVALIDE is not recommended.

Patients with Hepatic Impairment

No dosage adjustment is necessary in patients with hepatic impairment.

HOW SUPPLIED

AVAPRO® (irbesartan) is available as white to off-white biconvex oval tablets, debossed with a heart shape on one side and a portion of the NDC code on the other. Unit-of-use bottles contain 30, 90, or 500 tablets and blister packs contain 100 tablets, as follows:

	75 mg	150 mg	300 mg
Debossing	2771	2772	2773
Bottle of 30	0087-2771-31	0087-2772-31	0087-2773-31
Bottle of 90	0087-2771-32	0087-2772-32	0087-2773-32
Bottle of 500	—	0087-2772-15	0087-2773-15
Blister of 100	—	0087-2772-35	—

AVALIDE ® (irbesartan-hydrochlorothiazide) Tablets are peach, biconvex, and oval with a heart debossed on one side and 2775 or 2776 on the reverse, supplied as follows:

Irbesartan (mg)	HCTZ (mg)	NDC 0087-xxxx-xx for unit of use			
		Bottle of			Blister of
		30	90	500	100
150	12.5	2775–31	2775–32	2775–15	2775–35
300	12.5	2776–31	2776–32	2776–15	2776–35

Storage

Store at a temperature between 15° C and 30° C (59° F and 86° F) [See USP].

Distributed by:
Bristol-Myers Squibb Sanofi-Synthelabo Partnership
New York, NY 10016

1017108A8 (AVAPRO)
1030329A4 (AVALIDE)

Revised August 2002
B2-B001B-10-02

Bristol-Myers Squibb Company

sanofi~synthelabo

NOTES

NOTES

NOTES

NOTES

NOTES

NOTES